BLACK WOMEN SURVIVING SURVIVORSHIP

BLACK WOMEN SURVIVING SURVIVORSHIP

**Our Stories. Our Strength.
Our Survival Through Cancer.**

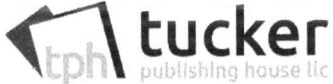

Copyright © 2025

Black Women Surviving Survivorship: Our Stories. Our Strength. Our Survival Through Cancer.

Authors: Judy Lawrence Lamb, Sabrina Thomas, Monica Poe, Nicole Lee, Sandra Ewing, Neicy Johnson, Renee Conley, Via May-Shephard, Lisa L. Gittens, LaToya Murphy, Valerie Wilder, Marisa Youngblood, and Tara Tucker.

All rights reserved. No part of this book may be reproduced, stored in a retrieval system, or transmitted in any form or by any means—electronic, mechanical, photocopying, recording, or otherwise—without the prior written permission of the publisher, except for brief quotations used in reviews or scholarly works.

Disclaimer: The information in this book is based on the authors' personal experiences and is not intended as medical advice. Readers should consult with qualified healthcare professionals regarding their individual health concerns.

Scripture Quotations: Unless otherwise noted, Scripture passages drawn from the King James Version (KJV) are in the public domain and may be quoted freely. Scripture quotations marked (NIV) are taken from The Holy Bible, New International Version®, © 1973, 1978, 1984, 2011 by Biblica, Inc.™ Used by permission of Zondervan. All rights reserved.

ISBN (Paperback): 979-8-9917761-9-6 (eBook): 978-1-970522-03-7

Publishing Services by: Tucker Publishing House, LLC
www.tuckerpublishinghouse.com

For permissions, bulk orders, or speaking engagements, contact: Tucker Publishing House, LLC admin@tuckerpublishinghouse.com

Cover design by Tucker Publishing House Interior design by Tucker Publishing House

Printed in the United States of America

First Edition

10 9 8 7 6 5 4 3 2 1

Contents

Introduction vii
Dear Sister ix
What You'll Find in These Pages x
In Loving Memory xi
Words from Ms. Kay's Daughter, Bria S. xiii

Stand, My Sister, Stand… 3
Authored By: Judy "Eve" Lawrence-Lamb
My Journey, My Faith: A Survivor's Story 21
Authored By: LaToya Murphy
Voice on the Altar 37
Authored By: Lisa L. Gittens
The Bald Eagle "Bald and Beautiful" 49
Authored By: Marisa Youngblood
My Journey Ain't Yours, and Yours Ain't Mine 63
Authored By: Monica Poe
Fought and Won! 75
Authored by: Neicy Johnson
Walk in Miracles 89
Authored By: Nicole Lee
My Journey through Endometrial/Uterine Cancer 101
Authored By: Renee Conley
Embracing Self-Care: A Guide to Thriving After Breast Cancer Treatment 111
Authored By: Sabrina Thomas

Thriving and Surviving 123
Authored by Sandra Ewing
He Did it For Me! Overcoming cancer with Jesus 133
Authored By: Valerie Wilder
Victory is Mine! 143
Authored By: Via May-Shephard
Embracing Change 155
Authored by: Tara Tucker

MEET THE AUTHORS 175-196
Meet Lisa! 175
Meet LaToya! 177
Meet Judy! 179
Meet Nicole! 180
Meet Via! 182
Meet Marisa! 184
Meet Sabrina! 186
Meet Renee! 187
Meet Monica! 188
Meet Neicy! 190
Meet Valerie! 192
Meet Sandra! 194
Meet Tara! 195
Epilogue: Your Story Continues 197
Resource 201

Introduction

The level of warfare that came up against this project was unmatched. There were so many times I wanted to quit. So many moments when I questioned whether I had made a mistake in starting it at all. The release date shifted three or four times—sometimes due to personal struggles, sometimes because of what our co-authors were facing.

I remember sitting at my computer, cursor blinking on a blank page, paralyzed by the weight of what we were trying to create. How do you compile stories about surviving when some of the storytellers are still fighting for their lives? How do you celebrate survivorship when the battle isn't over for everyone?

We lost a few of our sisters during this process. Their voices, which were meant to be woven into these pages, were silenced before they could share their full stories. Others are still fighting cancer, navigating second diagnoses, complications, and long-term side effects. The grief of that reality hit me in waves.

Cancer is a beast—a ruthless, consuming force that doesn't just change your body; it changes your entire life. It changes families, friendships, dreams, and futures. It leaves scars that go deeper than skin.

I mourned while creating *Black Women Surviving Survivorship: Our Stories. Our Strength. Our Survival Through Cancer.* There were days I couldn't open the document. Days when the memories were too raw, the grief too close. Days when I questioned whether I had the right to compile these stories when my own healing was still in process. But through it all, I thank God for healing—and for the grace I was given by these extraordinary women to process my pain while honoring theirs.

Each author in this collection brought her whole heart to these pages. They trusted me with their most vulnerable moments—their deepest fears, their greatest triumphs. They shared the parts of their stories that many people never see: the midnight terrors, the identity crises, the moments when hope felt impossible to find. They wrote through treatment fatigue, through grief, and through the ongoing reality that survivorship is not a finish line but a lifelong process.

Yes, there were delays—some within our control, many not. Medical emergencies interrupted deadlines. Family crises took precedence over manuscript reviews. Real life kept happening, because cancer survivors don't get to pause their entire existence to write about their experiences. But eventually, I knew it was time to pull up those big girl panties. I already had them on, but let's be real—they were slipping! Still, I pulled them up tight and pressed on. Because these stories—*our* stories—needed to be told.

Cancer touched each of us differently, yet in ways that felt hauntingly familiar. We all had to find a new normal. We all lost something—hair, breasts, energy, innocence, the luxury of assuming tomorrow was guaranteed. But in that loss, we discovered resilience we didn't know we had, a renewed sense of purpose that surprised us, and an unshakable faith that carried us through our darkest hours.

Dear Sister

I see you holding this book. Maybe you picked it up because the title caught your eye, or maybe someone placed it in your hands knowing you needed these particular voices today.

Here's what I want you to know before you turn another page: You don't have to be strong right now. You don't have to have it all figured out. You don't have to smile through the pain or pretend everything is fine when it isn't.

The women in these pages? They felt exactly what you're feeling—the fear, the anger, the confusion. The moments when faith felt impossible and hope seemed foolish.

But they also discovered something profound: you can be broken and blessed simultaneously. You can grieve what was while embracing what's becoming. You can question God and still trust Him.

"He heals the brokenhearted and binds up their wounds."
- Psalm 147:3 (ESV)

These aren't pretty stories with perfect endings. They're real stories from real women who bled courage onto these pages so you could find strength for your own journey. Some fought cancer multiple times. Others lost their voices, their identities, their sense of normalcy. All of them learned to thrive in spaces they never wanted to inhabit.

As you read, let their transparency give you permission to be honest about where you are. Let their victories remind you that surviving isn't just about making it through—it's about discovering who you become in the process.

You're not alone in this, Sister. Not today, not tomorrow, not ever.

What You'll Find in These Pages

This book is more than a collection of stories. *Black Women Surviving Survivorship* is a living testimony. A woven sisterhood. A declaration that we are more than what happened to our bodies. It is dedicated to every woman who has faced cancer—whether in her own body or through someone she loves. We see you. We honor you. We are surviving survivorship… together.

Welcome to your new beginning, beautiful. It's time to thrive.
Many blessings,

Coach Tara
Your favorite Shift Your Story Coach
#liveloveBEauthentic

In Loving Memory

Ramona Kaye Simons

Warrior. Woman of Faith. Forever in Our Hearts.

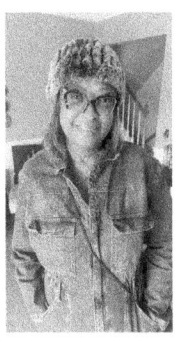

Though she never had the chance to write her chapter, Ramona Kaye Simons' story is still deeply a part of this book.

Her life was a testimony of strength, grace, and unwavering faith. She faced cancer with courage, refusing to be defined by her diagnosis. Ramona was more than a fighter—she was a light. A mother, a sister, a friend, and a woman who made others feel seen, loved, and supported even while walking through her own valley.

She was invited to be a part of this anthology because her voice mattered—and it still does. While the pages she might have written remain blank, her impact is anything but empty. Her absence left a space we cannot fill, but we honor her presence in every word written by her sisters in survivorship.

This two-page spread is for the story she didn't get to write, but one we all remember.

Her fight was not in vain.

Her love lives on.

Her courage continues to inspire.

"Many women do noble things, but you surpass them all."
— Proverbs 31:29

In Loving Memory

Words from Ms. Kay's Daughter, Bria S.

In Greek, the name Kaye means "pure". That's how I remember my Mom. Her joy, sweetness, and optimism were so authentic and pure; even after a life that wasn't always easy. My mom had the kind of optimism and hopefulness that was like a child untainted by the world. Even in the midst of a brutal cancer battle, she started every year believing, "This is going to be my year."

My own pessimistic nature sometimes thought it was foolish for her to think like that, but in the almost two years since she's been gone, God has already shown me that there were things she understood that I hadn't yet. Now I do. I say all of this to say that my mom was so excited to be a part of this anthology. She knew God had more for her to do, and she was willing and ready. She believed that her life was for others, and she lived that way until the end.

In one of our last conversations, she talked about going to her brother's doctor's appointment to advocate for him. She strongly believed that her story would touch the lives of others and inspire many. I'm still believing that for her. She left behind a legacy of love, joy, peace, patience, kindness, goodness, faithfulness, gentleness, and temperance. Like my pastor said when eulogizing her, she was a gift. A gift that my family and I don't go a day without missing. A gift that can never be replicated or replaced. I thank God for the greatest gift He could have given me.

I will love and miss her forever.
Bria

Dear Sister,

I am sharing my story with you because I want you to know that if you feel the world is crashing around you, you are not alone. It isn't easy feeling secluded from a life filled with peace, joy, goal setting, and making things happen to receiving a diagnosis that threatens to remove it all. It isn't easy seeing pain and hopelessness in the eyes of the people you love and who love you. It's hard to question your fate, having no idea what questions to ask. Silent tears are your only relief because you don't want to burden others, causing them to suffer as well. The burden you carry has your name on it; it's yours alone.

                                                Judy

Stand, My Sister, Stand...

Authored By: Judy "Eve" Lawrence-Lamb

It all began when I woke up from a peaceful sleep at 2 AM. I was led to touch my right breast. When I did, I discovered a large lump. I wasn't sure if it was something new or if it had always been there, hidden in plain sight like so many things we learn to live with until we can't ignore them anymore.

I fell back to sleep, but as soon as the sun rose, I went upstairs to tell my son, Allen. He was living with me at the time. I didn't hesitate because he had always been an early riser, and something about that lump felt urgent in the morning light.

I asked him to feel the lump. His response was immediate and clear: "Mama, this doesn't feel right. We need to have a doctor examine this."

From that moment, we were on a mission. We went to the doctor; he ordered a mammogram which showed a very large mass. From there, we were sent to have a biopsy done. My core family was there while the injections were being administered.

I find it interesting how when someone in authority shares their "knowledge" with us, we hang our hat on it. After the biopsy was completed, the technician looked at it and said, "This doesn't look bad at all." Those words gave me peace. So, we waited in peace for the results.

How naive we were to think that peace built on incomplete information could last.

Dreams Deferred but Not Denied

After encouraging the youth of my family to get a degree, I decided that by returning to school myself, I would be an example. I wanted to set a standard while holding myself accountable. I applied and was accepted at Norfolk State University in Virginia where I majored in English. I was 59 years old.

This wasn't just about education—this was about reclaiming the dreams I had deferred for decades while raising children and managing life's responsibilities. At 59, I felt like I was finally living for myself, not just for everyone else who needed me.

I woke up every morning in great anticipation of what the day would bring. I was very engaged in every aspect of my college experience. I was even the president of the honor society. Whenever there was a class project of any kind, I challenged my classmates to knock it out of the park by using their imagination and creativity.

Once in music appreciation, the project was the acknowledgment of various genres during different times throughout history. As part of my presentation, I used two of my granddaughters, Judea and Allena. They were dressed to represent a certain era. It was a hit! My professor told me that he was tempted to give me four A's. I felt as if God had put my life in reverse so that I could recapture the youth I had lost.

Little did I know that this season of recapturing youth would soon be interrupted by a test that would redefine everything I thought I knew about living.

The Phone Call That Changed Everything

One day after class, I was sitting in the student union waiting for my husband when my cell phone rang. I thought it was him letting me know that he had arrived. I was wrong.

It was the doctor informing me that my biopsy results were in and that I had cancer. He said more, but I had no idea what he was saying. All I remember is an overwhelming feeling of loneliness and disbelief.

The bustling student union around me seemed to fade into silence. Students laughing, talking, planning their futures—and here I was, wondering if I had a future at all. The contrast between their carefree energy and my sudden reality felt surreal.

Looking back, I wonder why he didn't check to see if I had any support as I was being given this life-changing news. A phone call in a public place, surrounded by strangers, is no way to learn that your life has just taken a dramatic turn.

When my husband came to pick me up, I told him what the doctor said, and he cried. The ride home was silent. I believe that both of us were at a loss for words. When we arrived home and as the garage door lifted, the first thing I saw was my son, Allen. I could see in his eyes that he already knew. I was trying to figure out how to tell him, and he was struggling with how he was going to tell me.

After sharing the news with my family, a plan of action went into effect. When you're facing a crisis, having people who love you enough to spring into action is a blessing beyond measure.

The Six-Month Sentence

When I was first diagnosed with Stage IV metastatic breast cancer, only my family and I were informed that I was looking at a possible six-month expiration date. It was devastating to think about how drastically my life would change and how little time I had to meet the goals I had set for myself.

Six months. Not even enough time to finish the semester, much less graduate. Not enough time to see another Christmas or watch my granddaughters grow into young women. Not enough time to finish the books I was reading or write the stories I had brewing in my heart.

The weight of that timeline felt crushing. How do you process the fact that everything you've planned, every dream you've deferred and finally started pursuing, might have to fit into less than half a year?

A Divine Direction

I made some life-altering decisions during this time. I was a member of Oak Grove Baptist Church for over 30 years. I loved serving in my church, and it was my home away from home. I was assistant church secretary, a member of the praise team, missionary circle president, founder and president of the First Lady's Day committee, choir member, president of the pastor's aide committee, member of the senior citizens committee, founder and director of the children's choir, praise dancer, member of the beautification committee, newsletter editor and writer, and on occasions, speaker. My church was my life.

Then one Wednesday evening at Bible study, I was led to request a meeting with my pastor afterward. As I sat among my church family, God showed me a vision of them suffering and hovering over me. I knew that this was about the cancer, but there was sort of a mystery for me as to why He was showing this to me.

However, as I climbed the stairs to meet with Pastor Copeland in his study, it began to make sense. If I were to remain there and be healed, the deliverance would be accredited to those around me rather than God. I had to be where there was no familiarity so that I would put all of my trust in Him.

Needless to say, the conversation that took place that night was difficult. My pastor was not only my under-shepherd; he was my friend of many years. How do you explain to someone who has shepherded you for three decades that God is calling you to leave for your own healing? How do you make someone understand that sometimes isolation is necessary for divine intervention?

But obedience to God sometimes requires us to make decisions that others can't understand, even when those decisions break our own hearts.

"Trust in the Lord with all your heart and lean not on your own understanding; in all your ways submit to him, and he will make your paths straight."
Proverbs 3:5-6 (ESV)

Finding a New Spiritual Home

Knowing that I needed to be a part of a Christian and progressive environment, I joined The Mount of Chesapeake. Of course, I had to do more there than warm the pews. I began working at the front desk. I also formed a senior citizen dance ministry. We loved hearing great Gospel music and choreographing. I adored my new pastor and really connected to his style of preaching. He showered my family and me with love. It didn't take long for me to feel right at home.

There was always something happening during the service to be a blessing to the people of God. I remember when I was very weak and had very little strength to do anything. A young woman who was a member there showed up at my door with cleaning supplies and a bucket. She cleaned my home from top to bottom. I cried as I watched her on her knees polishing every wooden piece of my bed. I was overwhelmed by her benevolence.

I emailed Pastor Brown to tell him about it. That Sunday, she was called to the front of the church, and she was showered with all denominations of dollar bills! It really blew me away when she came back to share a portion of her blessings with me.

Another great blessing was when my son was called to the pulpit by Pastor Brown. He shared with Allen that he was aware he was a single father with four children. He had a checkbook in his hand; he wrote a check for one month's rent.

Even though these beautiful acts may have seemed random, I know that they were ordained by God. This was confirmation that following God's direction to leave my familiar church home had been the right decision, even though it was painful.

There was never a service that someone wasn't blessed—be it with gas cards or monetary showers of love. I look back to that time and wonder where I would have been had I not left.

Eventually, my husband accepted a call from another church to become a deacon, and as his wife, I felt that it was only right for me to accompany him. He had supported me through everything that I did, and it was time for me to support him. He had never been offered a position in the church before, and I couldn't deny him this opportunity after he had been my rock through cancer.

Facing the Medical Battlefield

At our doctor's visit, I received the details of the diagnosis. There was no time to drag our feet; we had to get things in order. I was given options as to how we would move forward: "Did I only want one breast removed, or did I want both? When will I be able to have the surgery done? Which hospital did I prefer? Do I have anyone to assist me in getting my business in order? Did I want implants or reconstruction? How old was my grandma when she died from breast cancer?" So many questions!

Somehow, I found the strength to answer each one. Due to the cancer being metastatic, it was wise to have both breasts removed. I wanted to have the surgery done immediately; there was no point in holding on to something that was killing me. I wanted to go to a reputable hospital known for excellence in the field of oncology.

My business had been in order since October 1984 at the altar of Oak Grove Baptist Church when I accepted Jesus Christ as my Savior and Lord. Remembering how horrified my mother told me she was when she saw the results of her mother's mastectomy, I decided on implants. My grandmother was 45 when she lost the fight.

These decisions felt both monumental and strangely simple. When you're facing death, clarity has a way of cutting through all the noise and showing you what really matters.

Graduation Against All Odds

After everything that could be done was done surgically, I decided to return to campus. I had to wear a mask, but it was better than trying to keep up virtually. I needed to be present as an active participant.

Every day, my husband drove me to school, carried my books, walked me to class, helped me get seated, and waited in the car until I was ready to go to the next class. We did that until graduation day on May 4, 2013, which was the anniversary of the death of my firstborn who died in an automobile accident.

The symbolism of that date wasn't lost on me. Graduating on the anniversary of my son's death, while fighting for my own life, felt like God was weaving together themes of loss and triumph, endings and beginnings, in ways only He could orchestrate.

At graduation, I sat next to my youngest son, who was inspired by my determination. Even though he was a single father of three little girls and an adopted son, he felt that if I could meet the challenge, he could too. He graduated Summa cum laude with a 4.0; I graduated Magna cum laude with a 3.6.

The newspaper captured a beautiful picture of us giving each other a high five. The headline was "It was pomp and circumstances in spite of her circumstances." It was an enjoyable day of celebration, grilling at the park and enjoying family.

That graduation represented more than an academic achievement. It was proof that cancer couldn't stop me from finishing what I started. It was evidence that dreams deferred don't have to be dreams denied.

The Physical Battle

When chemotherapy began, I started seeing locks of my hair on the pillow each morning. I was forewarned that it would happen, but I was still very anticipatory about the impact it would have on me and my self-esteem.

I finally realized that I could allow fate to have the final say, or I could take matters into my own hands. I made an appointment with my hairdresser so that she could cut my hair. I remember some of my loved ones being with me as I watched my curls fall to the floor. I saw tears all around me as I felt my own running down my cheeks. I knew that this was only the beginning. When I returned home, my husband and my son shaved my head.

The first time I went out bald, I went to Lowe's. There was a little boy and girl looking at me, snickering. I have to admit that my feelings were hurt, but I didn't acknowledge those feelings or the children. When I returned home, I shared what had happened and how it made me feel.

My daughter Nichole said, "Mama, you can rock your bald head with some makeup and big hoop earrings!" I took her suggestion, and it worked! I don't know how others felt about it after that, but I know that it made me feel 100% better.

Sometimes the medicine we need comes from the people who love us most, wrapped in simple wisdom that transforms how we see ourselves.

A Business Built on Beauty

Speaking of makeup, my mind goes back to my Mary Kay Cosmetics days. I have always been known to be extra, and with this venture, I was no different. Before I was diagnosed, I was a Mary Kay beauty consultant. I was excited, and as with everything I did, I was all in. I went from independent beauty consultant to independent senior beauty consultant to star team builder to elite team leader to independent sales director within six months. Due to my love of watching people grow with me, I became an independent senior sales director soon after. I had earned two free cars and was well on my way to the pink Cadillac when cancer knocked on my door. However, I was blessed to see one of my offspring directors driving her free car.

My husband's dedication and commitment to me has always been phenomenal. He used to attend my skincare classes with me and give the ladies the Satin Hands treatment. He would bring my supplies in and set them up. He would "warm chatter" potential clients when I wasn't there to do it. Warm chatter is when you see a woman with great potential and ask if they are familiar with Mary Kay. He would continue by telling them that his wife was a beauty consultant and that he was sure I would love to meet them. They actually gave him their numbers! He would bring them to me.

It was at one of those classes that I met someone who years later became my bonus daughter. I planted the Mary Kay seed, and later she became a consultant herself. Her name is Latrese Carter, and we remain close to this very day. She introduced me to anthologies through connecting me with her anthologist friend, Cathy Staton. Before that, I was oblivious to the power of connections with authors sharing their authentic truth. Even though I had published books of my own, combined efforts of sharing our stories as a unit was beyond a blessing.

New Beginnings in Charlotte

Allen and I agreed that after graduation, it was time for a new beginning, so we decided to make Charlotte our home. We didn't waste any time; we moved in June of 2013. Allen went first to scout out the city before committing. Education standards and crime rate were our focus.

My mother and husband were both in their eighties at the time. Everyone wasn't on board initially because they felt that the move was too much for them. However, it was obvious that they were ready for a new beginning too because "When are we moving?" was a daily question.

When we moved to Charlotte, we moved to several different homes trying to find the right fit. It was never stressful for us. My husband, mother, and I were spared the stress of moving; my kids took care of everything. I guess change is a treat when the alternative is to sit in a rocking chair or on a porch swing, waiting for God to call our names.

We even tried multigenerational living until Allen received a promotion that called for him to relocate to Georgia. With a few expected hiccups, it was a beautiful blend of ages. It was vibrancy and wisdom under one roof. As a result of our experience together, I wrote a children's book entitled "Under One Roof…Multigenerational Living and Loving." The grandson of a friend who loved to draw was one of my illustrators.

Finding Purpose in Teaching

When we moved to Charlotte, I became a substitute teacher for an elementary school. I loved it, but unfortunately, I had to take the children outside for recess. With one of the medications I took, I couldn't be exposed to the sun, so I tried middle school. I was silently triggered every day by the hormones. Visions of my children at that age reminded me that I didn't want to revisit those days. I took my son's advice and began taking assignments for high school.

When I first walked through the doors of Providence Sr. High School, I was somewhat intimidated. The students were taller than me; they were adults! My first thought was "What have I gotten myself into now?!" However, it didn't take me long to realize that I had made a very wise decision.

They called me "Ms. J." I became a go-to person for an encouraging boost, whether personal or academic. The classes that were labeled as "bad" somehow were always on their best behavior for me. Some of them began calling me "Grandma." It wasn't odd to hear a blonde-haired and blue-eyed kid screaming across the lunchroom, "Hey Grandma!" I was surprised to learn that many of them didn't have grandmothers in their lives.

They were always doing sweet little "pink" things for me in honor of my survivorship. Pink ribbons. Pink pictures. Pink shoelaces. Pink sweatshirts. These teenagers, who the system had labeled as problematic, saw me as someone worth honoring and protecting.

The Special Assignment

One day, I was called to the office by the principal. She told me that they had lost a teacher from the special needs class. She wanted to know if I was interested in a long-term substitute position. Even though I loved my high school students, I was drawn to the special needs kids when they were on the track or in the cafeteria. I said "Yes."

On my first day, a little 15-year-old girl named Megan caught my attention. She didn't mingle with the rest of the class; she was in her own little world. She wouldn't make eye contact with me when I spoke to her. I got the impression that she would rather not be bothered, but I didn't give up.

Before I knew it, Megan would hop up when she saw me come through the door. She would grab my hand and guide me to the door to go on our daily walks. We would either go to the track or around the hallways of the school.

When COVID invaded us, I considered my lingering health issues and discontinued my assignment there. Megan's parents asked if I would consider getting trained to homeschool her because they had the same concerns for her. That was nine years ago.

She is now 25 years old, and even though she is unable to speak, her love for me is spoken through her eyes—the same eyes that wouldn't meet mine 10 years ago. Her touch when she guides me to what she wants to do, like taking a walk, or what she wants to eat or drink by guiding me to the refrigerator. Her silent love for me drowns out the high frequencies of insincere spoken love.

Before William stopped driving, we would pick her up and take her home every day. I had some strange side effects from the chemotherapy treatments and hadn't driven for almost 12 years. I get anxious when cars are on the opposite side of the road. They look as if they're headed straight toward me. But God is good!

I am employed at 75, doing what I love to do, being loved by this now young woman, having her dropped off in the morning and picked up at night, taking leisurely walks and not having to fight traffic. Nobody but God could bless like that. Her parents and I have a beautiful relationship. I don't have to take off work or call off when I need to take a trip; where I go, Megan goes. It doesn't matter whether it's New York City, Myrtle Beach, Hilton Head, Louisiana, or any place in between.

Here I am today with only memories of the man who stood with me for 31 years throughout every season of my life. He went home to be with the Lord on Saturday, November 29, 2025. His last word before crossing over was "Judy." He left behind a legacy of strength and empowerment. Rest in peace my earthly lord and soulmate—William Lamb.

The Valley and Mountain Seasons

I don't want to give the impression that since that day in the student union, life has been a bed of roses. There were some mountains, but I've had a lion's share of valleys. What I found out, though, is that there was some refining, restoration, renewing, and rewards in the valley.

It was in the valleys that poems, sermons, song lyrics, books, plays, and creative visions were conceived. Then God would deliver me to the mountain so that I could give birth to that which was conceived in the valley.

My life has been filled with experiences in both the valleys and the mountains, but it is for sure that God never forsook me. Even when I didn't feel His presence, looking back, I know He was that Present Help He promised to be.

---

*"God is our refuge and strength,
an ever-present help in trouble."*
Psalm 46:1 (ESV)

The Grandma Judy Eve Ministry

There's one thing that comes natural to me, and that is being a grandma, which is why I took on the character "Grandma Judy Eve." I dress up in my vintage dress, white apron, pearls, and grey wig. I love going to children's events, schools, and parks to read to the children. It is as much a blessing for me as it is for them.

This ministry grew out of my understanding that children need to see older adults who are vibrant, engaged, and full of stories. In a world where families are often scattered and generations don't always connect, I wanted to be a bridge between young and old, sharing wisdom through story and presence.

The Moment of Truth

There was one time that I felt sorry for myself. The children were off to school. Allen was out of sight. William was watching the news. Mama, who was staying with me to help out, was in her bedroom. I was lying in the same spot on that green leather sofa in our family room.

Suddenly I became angry and frustrated. I grabbed hold of the tubes hanging from the incisions and went in search of Allen. I blasted him for leaving me alone with horrifying thoughts of my disfigurement. I snatched my shirt up to expose my breasts. "How would you like it if this had happened to you?!" I shouted.

I didn't expect his response. "They actually look pretty good, Mama."

At the time, I didn't know that Allen had just returned from a long prayerful walk around the neighborhood on my behalf. He told me that as he was praying, he stopped and began laughing. He was expressing the joy of the message he received from the Holy Spirit telling him that I was going to be all right.

My Jamie and my Nichole weren't as strong as Allen. I believe they actually avoided me because it was too painful for them. One night, I was sitting in the middle of my bed surrounded by my family. I told them that if I didn't make it, it wouldn't be because I didn't try. My second granddaughter, Adrienne, told me that I couldn't die because I had to dance for God. I will never forget that.

I assured them that I was in a win-win situation. If I survived, I won. If God took me home, I won.

The Harvest Season

Now here I am—a little over a decade later. This isn't the season to plant in the heat of the day. I believe with all of my heart that God canceled my expiration date because He wants me to enjoy a season of harvest—harvest that goes beyond financial gain and social status.

It's a harvest of being a mother, grandmother, and great-grandmother. It's a harvest of still listening to music, laughing, and talking with my 96-year-old mother. It's a harvest of still being married to a man who honors me and loves me with all of his heart. It's a harvest of having a reasonable portion of health. It's a harvest of being in my right mind and able to use my gifts. It's a harvest of being gainfully employed at 75 while fulfilling my purpose. It's a harvest of my being able to share with you that there's hope.

That six-month prognosis became more than a decade of productive, purposeful living. The doctors were wrong about my timeline, but God was right about His plans for me.

The Secret to Survival

Cancer may have changed the life we once knew, but we still have life, and that's why we still have hope. The reason that we're here is because our assignments haven't been completed. God has more in store for us, and we must not faint.

We can aspire to be like Paul and whatever state we find ourselves in, we must be content. We are not privy to God's plan, but we must trust it. I've got a feeling that it's not all about the pie in the sky or walking around Heaven all day. I believe God has some rewards for us here on earth. In order that He be glorified, He wants some witnesses—witnesses that have not yet come to know Him, witnesses whose eyes will be opened.

When you're in the army of the Lord and on the battlefield, you have to endure spiritual boot camp. It's not to break you; it's to mold and make you. You were fearfully and wonderfully created in the image of God, so trust that you were fully equipped with the whole armor of God. Defeat is not an option. Giving up or in is not an option. Weeping as the world weeps is not an option. The mindset that your suffering is a result of something you've done is not an option.

There is only one option. That option is to trust God and never doubt that He will surely bring you out.

Why I'm Still Here

Why am I still here? I'm still here because through it all, I learned to trust God. When those "Job-like" spirits arrived at my door, they were thanked for coming but never got to see me.

We continued to laugh when things were funny even though we cried when they weren't. I had a friend, Rita, who regularly brought food to my home from Boston Market. Even though I couldn't eat most of the time, I was blessed that my family experienced some normalcy.

Every morning upon waking up, I thanked God that I was given another day of brand-new mercy. My eyes were two gifts that He opened day after day.

If the question was asked of me, "What was the secret to your survival?" my answer would be emphatic: "I found power in spending time with positive people." Negativity is not only draining; it's debilitating. Many people mean well but are unable to see valley blessings. They can't praise God while the problem still exists. They have to wait for the battle to be over before celebrating the victory.

Not so with me. I have come to realize that when we praise God in advance, it is a testament of our faith. It is a rejection of defeat and an expression of victory.

"Weeping may endure for a night, but joy comes in the morning."
Psalm 30:5 (ESV)

Stand, My Sister, Stand

Do not, my sister, go quietly into the night. Having done all to stand, stand! There is no testimony without a test.

You may be facing your own six-month prognosis. You may be sitting in a doctor's office receiving news that threatens to steal your future. You may be wondering how you'll find the strength to fight, the faith to believe, the courage to hope.

Let me tell you what I learned: God's timeline is not the doctor's timeline. His plan is not limited by medical prognoses. His power is not constrained by statistics or survival rates.

Stand in your truth. Stand in your faith. Stand in the knowledge that you were created for such a time as this, and your story is not over until God says it's over.

The harvest season is coming, sister. The best is yet to be.

"Therefore, my dear brothers and sisters, stand firm. Let nothing move you. Always give yourselves fully to the work of the Lord, because you know that your labor in the Lord is not in vain."
1 Corinthians 15:58 (ESV)

Stand, my sister, stand.

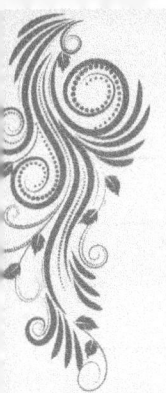

If the question was asked of me "What was the secret to your survival?" My answer would be emphatic..." I found power in spending time with positive people." Negativity is not only draining; it's debilitating. Many people mean well but are unable to see valley blessings. They can't praise God while the problem still exists. They have to wait for the battle to be over before celebrating the victory. Not so with me. I have come to realize that when we praise God in advance, it is a testament of our faith. It is a rejection of defeat and an expression of victory.

Judy Eve Lawrence Lamb

My Dear Sister,

I wrote this chapter just for you. You need to know that no matter what you are faced with, there is greater for you and you will get through this. My testimony was about cancer. Your testimony may not be my testimony, but the good news is, we all have a testimony. And when you have a testimony, that means you passed the test. I want to encourage you that God is still performing miracles and He is not short concerning His promises. What He promised you, He will bring it to past. Continue to walk by faith and don't be moved by what you see, feel or hear. Stand firm on God's Word and don't doubt, you too will see the manifestation of His Word. He is able and He won't fail!!!

Philippians 4:13 declares, "You can do anything through Christ, who gives you strength."

Blessings,
LaToya

My Journey, My Faith: A Survivor's Story

Authored By: LaToya Murphy

It was 2012, and all was going well until I heard the word CANCER! It seemed like the wind was knocked out of me, and questions flooded my mind:

"Why me?" "What did I do to deserve this?" "Is God mad at me?" "Did I do something wrong?"

I mean, I'm only 33 years old. I'm too young to have this, according to the doctors. I'm not supposed to get a mammogram until I'm 40 years old.

"What am I supposed to do now?" "Am I going to die?"

These and more were the questions that entered my mind. As you can imagine, I was experiencing a fear that I just could not explain.

But let me tell you how it all began.

After leaving work and rushing home to relax and eat, I began to cook. While waiting for the food to finish, I decided to have a snack. As I was sitting on the couch, watching television, swinging my feet, and eating my favorite cookies, a crumb fell on my shirt near my left breast.

Such a simple thing—a cookie crumb. Who would have thought that this tiny moment would change the entire trajectory of my life?

I began to wipe the crumb away, and the next thing I knew, I came to a complete stop. My hand paused on my left breast. It felt different. It was a hard knot. I jumped up off the couch, and my hand was still rubbing across my left breast. The thumping of my heartbeat got faster and faster. I ran to my bedroom.

Terror. That's the only word that describes what I felt in that moment. Pure terror.

At the time, I was married, and I called for my husband. He came around the corner and asked, "Toya, what is wrong?"

I grabbed his hand and asked him to feel the knot on my chest. At first, he seemed happy as he rested his hand on my chest, excitement gleaming in his eyes. But his smile quickly faded, replaced by a frown.

He, too, felt the knot and withdrew his hand abruptly. "What is that?" he asked.

I replied, "I don't know, and I'm scared."

With a weird look in his eyes, he tried to encourage me by saying, "It's probably nothing to worry about."

Even though I wanted to believe him—oh, how I wanted to believe him—I couldn't shake the feeling of unease. I quickly grabbed my cell phone, realizing I only had a few minutes before the doctor's office closed for the day. Nervously, I dialed the number. After a few rings, a nurse answered. I hurriedly explained who I was and what I had just experienced. She calmly scheduled an appointment for me to see the doctor the very next day.

That night was the longest night of my life. My mind raced with possibilities, each one scarier than the last. Sleep felt impossible when your brain won't stop creating worst-case scenarios.

The Longest Wait

When morning came, I got up, got dressed, and prepared to see my doctor. Anxiety gripped me, tightening its hold with every passing minute. By the time I arrived and sat in the lobby waiting to be called, my nerves were through the roof.

Finally, I heard my name. I stood up and followed the nurse to the exam room, where she calmly instructed me to undress from the waist up. Sitting there, waiting for the doctor to come in, I felt tears streaming down my face. I couldn't help it—the fear was overwhelming.

When the doctor finally entered the room, it was clear from his expression that he could see the worry etched on my face. He assured me by saying, "You should have nothing to worry about."

The doctor began examining my left breast and suggested doing a needle biopsy right away. He calmly explained the procedure, showing me the long needle he was about to use. As he prepared to insert it into my chest, he told me to relax as much as I could. I assured him I wasn't afraid of needles and was okay for the moment.

But looking back, I wasn't okay. I was terrified. I just didn't know how to express it.

When the procedure was finished, he instructed me to get dressed and said he would call with the results in a week. I nodded slowly and said, "Okay." He reassured me not to worry, and I wanted to believe him. After all, he was the doctor—surely, he would know.

I left the office holding on to his words, hoping they would be enough to ease my growing fear. But hope and fear were wrestling in my heart, and I wasn't sure which one would win.

The Phone Call That Stopped Time

As each day passed—which felt like an eternity—it finally became the week I had been waiting for. I held on to the hope that I'd receive good news. I was standing in my classroom, working with students, when my phone rang. I stared at it for a moment and saw that it was the doctor's office calling. My heartbeat raced so fast, it felt like it was pounding in my toes.

"Hello?" I answered, my voice shaky.

"Hi, is this LaToya?" the doctor's voice asked.

"Yes, this is LaToya," I replied, trying to keep calm.

"This is Dr. S. I've got your results back. There are some cancer cells, so we need you to come back to the office to discuss the next steps. I wanted to call you personally to tell you the news."

Cancer cells. The words hit me like a physical blow.

The moment he spoke those words, it felt like my world came to a complete stop, and everything slowed down. I froze for a second, the tears already streaming down my face.

"Okay, okay, thank you," I said, my voice barely a whisper.

I hung up the phone, and before I even realized it, I was running out of the room, screaming, "NO!" I dashed down the hall, completely forgetting I had a classroom full of students who needed me. In that moment, I wasn't a teacher anymore—I was just a terrified woman who had just received news that felt like a death sentence.

The school counselor was coming down the hall, whom I affectionately called my "work mom." She reached out and grabbed me and began to ask what was wrong. I could only utter the words, "cancer."

She asked, "Who has cancer?"

I replied, "Me! The doctor said I had cancer!"

She asked, "So do you think you're going to die?"

I hunched my shoulders because I didn't know. I honestly didn't know.

The Room Where Faith Was Born

She reminded me that I should trust God and told me to go into the empty room across the hall. Her words to me were words I will never forget: "Have your pity party for a few minutes, but when you come out of that room, you better remember who you are and whose you are. Trust the God that you serve and believe you are going to be alright. You have a calling on your life, and He is not going to let you die like this."

I hugged her, and I walked into that room.

While in the room, I cried. My heart was heavy with so many questions for God. Why now? Why me? What was I supposed to do with this news? But in that moment of desperation, I remembered the word of knowledge my pastor spoke each week. The "Confessions of Faith" that he would have us say, week after week. I used to question why we repeated them so often, but now, at this moment, I finally understood their purpose.

The very scriptures I got tired of repeating, I now needed desperately.

My pastor always encouraged us to say those scriptures until they became a part of our daily walk, knowing we would one day need them. He often said, "What's in us will eventually come out of us." As I dried my tears, I walked out of that room with a faith I had read about in the Bible all these years but never fully experienced. I felt a surge of strength as I reflected on those scriptures.

Standing in the hallway was my "work mom," who is also a pastor's wife. She looked at me with a warm smile and said, "Now, that's what I want to see. I know you'll be just fine."

I hugged her tightly, feeling reassured, and made my way back to the classroom, suddenly realizing I had completely forgotten where I was... and those poor students! To this day, I sincerely apologize for that moment of abandonment. But sometimes, crisis strips away everything except what's essential, and in that moment, I had to find my faith before I could help anyone else.

> *"Trust in the Lord with all your heart and lean not on your own understanding; in all your ways submit to him, and he will make your paths straight."*
> **Proverbs 3:5-6 (ESV)**

The Decision to Fight with Faith

Things moved quickly since my breast cancer diagnosis—Stage 2B carcinoma in my left breast. I underwent numerous surgeries, scans, X-rays, and tests—so many that I lost count. I met several doctors I would be seeing throughout this process. It had been a month, and my oncologist told me I needed to undergo six rounds of chemotherapy.

I wasn't sure what to expect, but I made a decision that would define my entire cancer journey: I was going to walk by faith and not by sight.

To this day, I haven't shared the diagnosis with anyone in my family initially. I only confided in a few pastor friends who were faith believers and would trust God with me. Every day, I carried a copy of the healing scriptures and confessions of faith my pastor gave us at church.

This wasn't because I didn't love my family or trust them. It was because I knew that in this battle, I needed to surround myself only with voices that would strengthen my faith, not weaken it. I only wanted people around me who spoke positively, who believed in the Word of God, and who would stand in faith on my behalf. There was no room in my life for doubters, naysayers, or those with uncertainties.

It came down to trusting God or nothing. My life was truly in His hands, and that's where I needed to keep my focus.

Some people might think this approach was extreme, but when you're fighting for your life, you have to be strategic about what you allow into your atmosphere. Faith is fragile when it's being tested, and I couldn't afford to let doubt creep in through well-meaning but fear-filled voices.

When the Doctor Became a Believer

With my scriptures in hand, I reached chemotherapy round three. That day, my oncologist smiled and said to me, "You've convinced me that a positive attitude can kill cancer."

He had noticed how I'd come to each appointment, smiling and joking, always carrying my scriptures—what I called my "buddies." He looked at my blood work and medical charts and told me how proud he was of me.

I confidently told him, "My hair is not going to fall out."

He laughed and said it would after the third round of chemo.

I laughed too and told him that God wouldn't allow my hair to fall out.

Well, within a few days, it started shedding heavily. I laughed and told God, "You're funny." My then-husband shaved my head bald. It was difficult and different, but my faith only grew stronger. Sometimes God's plan doesn't match our expectations, but that doesn't mean He's not working on our behalf.

I knew that God had a calling on my life, but I had never answered it until that moment. Easter was approaching fast, and I answered my calling, preaching my first sermon on a Saturday, just days after chemo that Monday.

Standing in My Purpose

I remember that Easter Saturday like it was yesterday. I sat in the church office, listening to the service and feeling the energy of the audience. A few close friends helped me with my makeup and hair—what little I had left. They walked with me as I made my way to the pulpit. My heart raced, and hot flashes flared up, but I could hear the clapping and cheering from my family and friends who came from all over to support me.

It felt so natural for me to be there in that moment, surrounded by my supporters. The time had come for me to stand at the sacred desk and encourage others with the Word of God, even though I needed encouragement myself.

My short introduction turned into a song: "I am grateful for the things that You have done..." Tears filled everyone's eyes, and praise exploded in the building. As I continued to sing, the song encouraged me more than anyone else.

In the middle of my sermon, I was encouraged to release my testimony about having cancer. You could hear a pin drop on the carpet. It got so quiet in the church, and I could see friends and family begin to cry as they were in disbelief. No one except the few people I told at the beginning knew I had cancer until that very moment.

I had to say something because the hotter I got, the more I began to sweat, and my wig was slipping off.

Oh, the conversations that happened at that moment. "What?" "Are you serious?" "She has cancer?" "Did you know?"

I reminded them not to feel sorry for me. I told them I would be "just fine." The boldness came over me as I began to recite the scriptures that I carried around every day, confessing my healing. I was seeing the results as I used them, and I wanted them to understand that the Word was working for me, and it could work for them too if they believed.

As the service came to an end and I greeted everyone, I was overwhelmed by the love shown for me that day. I left that place feeling complete and knowing God was smiling on me.

Easter Revelations

It was Easter, and after church, we gathered at my parents' house to eat and fellowship. It was there that I finally opened up to my immediate family about my cancer journey so far.

There was a mix of emotions in the room that day. My family was shocked, unable to believe that I had gone through all of this without telling them. Some were hurt that I hadn't confided in them. Others were amazed at how I had handled it. All of them were scared.

I explained to them that God had placed me on a path where I had to trust Him completely, and for that season, I couldn't tell anyone. I had to avoid hearing negativity, doubt, and questions that could shake my faith.

My mother cried and said she wished she could have been there for me. I told her she was—through the foundation of faith she had given me growing up.

My siblings wanted to know how they could help now. I told them the best thing they could do was speak life over me and trust God with me.

I want to take a moment to encourage you: Sometimes, when you're going through a trial, you can't speak about your test—you just have to trust the tester. God will place us in situations where He's testing us to see if He can trust us to believe what He says.

One of my favorite confessions is: "I do follow the good shepherd, and I know His voice. The voice of a stranger I will not follow. Therefore, I confess that in my pathway is life, and there is no death."

I stood on that confession and believed it, holding on to it until I saw the evidence.

The Victory Lap

I continued my chemotherapy, faithfully going through all six rounds of treatments. Each session was a step closer to victory, though some days it felt more like endurance than triumph.

Then came the moment I had been waiting for:

"Good news, LaToya! This will be your last chemo treatment. Everything went according to plan, and I'm so excited for you," said the oncologist.

The joy that flooded my heart was indescribable as tears streamed down my face. All I could say was, "Thank you, God, for loving me enough to heal me."

A few weeks later, I was referred to the radiologist and scheduled my appointment. I'd heard negative things about radiation, but I continued to trust God.

The day of my appointment, I saw the radiologist, and these were her words: "Hi, LaToya. I was just looking at your charts. I see you have completed chemotherapy. Congratulations! The next step is radiation when referred by your doctor."

She took off her glasses that were lying on the tip of her nose and slid them back over her hair. These were her words: "Well, I am looking at your paperwork, and I'm going to tell you the truth. If I were to do radiation on you, it would be a waste of my time and yours. Again, congratulations. Glad I could not help you. You may leave."

Standing there in amazement, I asked her to repeat what she said.

She smiled and said, "Bye, LaToya. You heard me correctly."

I said my thanks and told her this was great news. I ran out of her office and dashed to the hallway without looking back. While in the hallway, I burst into tears and told God thank you as I leaped and jumped.

A man walking by said to me, "You must have some great news."

I said, "Sir, if you only knew. I don't have time to tell you, but I'm getting out of here."

He laughed and said, "Okay," as I quickly exited the building and ran to my car.

When I walked through those sliding doors, I paused briefly and took a deep breath. It felt like I could breathe again after receiving the news. I threw my hands up as a sign of thank you to God and proceeded to get in my car.

---

*"He sent out his word and healed them;
he rescued them from the grave."*
Psalm 107:20 (ESV)

Surgery and Setbacks

A few weeks went by, leading to my scheduled surgery. I decided to call the doctor's office and ask about a surgery date for breast removal and reconstruction. I was given a choice to remove one or both. So I decided to do both, which is called bilateral reconstruction, because I didn't want to risk the chance of the cancer coming back.

Of course, I trusted God, but I had to use wisdom. People always question me about why I removed both instead of one. I'd laugh and say, "The Bible tells us to not be unequally yoked."

At this point, if I believe the Word, I must be all in. And I was definitely all in.

But as I waited for the scheduler to schedule my surgery date, I started getting a little nervous. Negative thoughts about what could possibly go wrong during surgery began creeping in. I chuckled a little and started thinking about my healing scriptures. Remembering those scriptures grabbed my negative thoughts, and I started to calm down while waiting for a confirmed date.

What's funny is that the surgery scheduler told me I was such a great patient that they completely forgot about me. At first, I was confused, but then I was grateful to hear those words. I'm sure that doesn't happen often, so I knew it was God working on my behalf.

Well, surgery arrived, and I had my immediate family with me for support. I was nervous and excited at the same time. This was a day that I couldn't have my "buddies" with me—the physical scriptures I carried. But the Word I had hidden in my heart was still there.

You see, I had repeated those scriptures so much they became a part of me. I didn't need the paper anymore; it was in my heart.

Surgery was now over, and I was in the ICU. When I woke up, all I could see was my family looking at me through the glass windows. As the nurses allowed them to come in two at a time, I noticed their worried expressions.

With what little strength I had, I asked them what was wrong. They told me that my surgery had lasted much longer than expected. What was supposed to be a 6-to-8-hour procedure ended up taking more than 12 hours. The doctors had struggled with the tissue on my left side, and they didn't know what was going on until the surgeon finally came out and explained.

This caused a lot of fear for my family. As they were walking out of my room, my right side went numb, and the alarms on the machines began blaring. Panic set in as the nurses rushed in to assist. Fear overwhelmed me as they moved me around and inserted tubes into my nose. They repeatedly asked if I was okay, and I shook my head yes, though I wasn't entirely sure.

The only thing that came to mind was the story in the Bible about King Hezekiah turning his face to the wall and praying to the Lord. I couldn't let my faith die at that moment, so I decided to do the same. I whispered, "Jesus" over and over.

Immediately, the alarms stopped, and everything calmed down. The nurses looked at each other, confused, unsure of what had just happened. I couldn't help but smirk because I knew God had heard me.

Before they exited the room, they asked once more if I was okay. I told them that I was.

Recovery and Complications

The next day, I was moved to a regular room because my vitals were looking good. However, I kept complaining about the burning sensation in my right arm. Each time I mentioned it, the nurses flushed out the IV, but they never adjusted or removed it, and the discomfort only increased.

I informed them every time they came in to check my vitals or surgery site, but they seemed more focused on my left breast, where my body was rejecting the tissue and the readings on the machine weren't coming through. After several unsuccessful readings, the doctors decided to remove the tissue from my left breast and insert a tissue expander. I was scheduled for surgery the very next day.

To say I was nervous is an understatement. Surgery so soon after the first one wasn't part of my plan. But God had a plan, and the surgery went smoothly. I stayed in the hospital for about two weeks while my family took turns staying with me until I was discharged.

For a month, I wore the tissue expander, and then it was surgery time again—expander out, silicone in. During my recovery, I began noticing that my right arm hurt more than ever. When the nurse removed the IV, my right arm was completely stiff, and I couldn't move it at all. It was stuck in a folded position, and I couldn't move it.

This was terrifying. Here I was, celebrating victory over cancer, only to discover that the treatment had caused another problem entirely.

I was recovering from surgery and being referred to a physical therapist, but through it all, I kept trusting God in the process. After four months of intensive therapy, my arm slowly began to move. The Word was still working for me, even when my circumstances looked discouraging.

Twelve Years of Faithfulness

Today, I am a 12-year breast cancer survivor. In March 2023, my oncologist released me with a clean bill of health. He told me, "Well, LaToya, everything looks great, and I'm so proud of your progress. I no longer need to see you. It feels like I'm losing a daughter. This has been a journey, but I have to release you. I'm here if you need me. Take care of yourself."

It was a bittersweet moment, but I'm grateful to be a living testimony of God's healing power. My doctor removed me from Tamoxifen, the chemo pill I took for ten years as a precaution after chemotherapy. God is still performing miracles.

I have no side effects, and I never got sick during the entire process. God truly favored me.

But the journey isn't over.

The Plot Twist

UH OH! Guess what I found out? All of my surgeries from 12 years ago were done incorrectly. I now need to undergo bilateral surgery again to correct the mistakes. According to the new breast surgeon, it will take several surgeries to fix it.

When I first heard this news, I'll admit I felt a moment of "Really, God? Again?" But then I remembered who I am and whose I am. I remembered that the same God who brought me through the first time is still faithful. I remembered that I am not just a survivor—I am an overcomer.

I can't wait to share this next chapter of my story with you. A survivor is still surviving! I still trust God!

This revelation reminded me that our faith journey is ongoing. Just when we think we've reached the finish line, God sometimes reveals that there's more race to run. But I'm not discouraged—I'm encouraged! Because if He brought me through once, He can bring me through again.

> *"Being confident of this, that he who began a good work in you will carry it on to completion until the day of Christ Jesus."*
> **Philippians 1:6 (ESV)**

The Power of the Word

Do you want to have the same testimony? Will you trust that God can heal you too? Will you allow the Word to work for you?

Let me encourage you to trust Him and stand on His promises. You can overcome sickness and disease, just as I did. Believe and receive the healing that God has for you.

The gift of song kept me encouraged throughout, and I never stopped singing. I would remind others that no matter what test you face, never stop using your gifts. It will keep you encouraged until you've passed the test. Believe me, it works.

Here are the healing scriptures that carried me through my journey:

Healing Scriptures

Jesus is the Lord of my life. Sickness and disease have no power over me. I am forgiven and free from sin and guilt. I am dead to sin and alive to righteousness. *Colossians 1:21, 22*

Jesus bore my sins in His Body on the tree; therefore I am dead to sin and alive unto God and by His stripes I am healed and made whole. *1 Peter 2:24; Romans 6:11; 2 Corinthians 5:21*

Jesus bore my sickness and carried my pain. Therefore I give no place to sickness or pain. For God sent His Word and healed me. *Psalm 107:20*

No evil will befall me, neither shall any plague come near my dwelling. For You have given Your angels charge over me. They keep me in all my ways. In my pathway is life, healing and health. *Psalm 91:10,11; Proverbs 12:28*

Jesus took my infirmities and bore my sicknesses. Therefore I refuse to allow sickness to dominate my body. The Life of God flows within me bringing healing to every fiber of my being. *Matthew 8:17; John 6:63*

My body is the temple of the Holy Spirit. I make a demand on my body to release the right chemicals. My body is in perfect chemical balance. My pancreas secretes the proper amount of insulin for life and health. *1 Corinthians 6:19*

Growths and tumors have no right to my body. They are a thing of the past for I am delivered from the authority of darkness. *Colossians 1:13,14*

Every organ and tissue of my body functions in the perfection that God created it to function. I forbid any malfunction in my body in Jesus' Name. *Genesis 1:28,31*

Your Word is manifest in my body, causing growths to disappear. Arthritis is a thing of the past. I make a demand on my bones and joints to function properly in Jesus' Name. *Mark 11:23; Matthew 17:20*

Thank You Father that I have a strong heart. My heart beats with the rhythm of life. My blood flows to every cell of my body restoring life and health abundantly. *Proverbs 12:14; 14:30*

I command my blood cells to destroy every disease, germ and virus that tries to inhabit my body. I command every cell of my body to be normal in Jesus' Name. *Romans 5:17; Luke 17:6*

I make a demand on my joints to function perfectly. There will be no pain or swelling in my joints. My joints refuse to allow anything that will hurt or destroy their normal function. *Proverbs 17:22*

You have forgiven all my iniquities; You have healed all my diseases; You have redeemed my life from destruction; You have satisfied my mouth with good things so that my youth is renewed as the eagles. *Psalm 103:2-5*

You have given me abundant life. I receive that life through Your Word and it flows to every organ of my body bringing healing and health. *John 10:10; John 6:63*

I am redeemed from the curse. Galatians 3:13 is flowing in my bloodstream. It flows to every cell of my body, restoring life and health. *Mark 11:23; Luke 17:6*

My affliction will leave and not come back again. *Nahum 1:9*

Make these words a part of your daily life and apply them to your daily living.

This is how I survived. Now, you can too!

My Dear Sister,

I'm writing this to you because I want you to know that your beauty reaches beyond what people or even what you can see with the naked eye. You are strong. You are resilient. You are a survivor.

I struggled and still do today sometimes with what I look like. My confidence is not the greatest, but I'm happy to be alive. I remember that I'm more than what I see when I look in the mirror. I hope that you can see that too. Much love to you. We are children of God, made in His image, and that's a BEAUTIFUL thing.

Lisa

Voice on the Altar

Authored By: Lisa L. Gittens

"I will bless the Lord at all times, and His praise shall continually be in my mouth. God, I will praise you in every situation."
I don't think we realize that when we make those declarations, they will come back around and that we will be tested. I've said this so many times and meant it. I still mean it today. God has been so good, so why *would I not praise Him? Why would I not serve Him? Why would I not give Him my life and my heart?*

But I was severely tested. This test changed my life forever and challenged everything I thought I knew about praising God "in every situation."

The Discovery

In 2020, I felt this small lump at the bottom of my mouth, right at the center. However, I wasn't immediately concerned. I didn't think about what it could be. I *never* thought it would be cancer.

At first, I thought it was one of those cold sores that you get in your mouth, so I did the home remedy of rinsing my mouth with salt and water, thinking that it would help it go down. Unfortunately, that didn't work. It started to get bigger and bigger, and I got used to it being there.

Looking back, I realize how dangerous it is to "get used to" something wrong in your body. We adapt, we normalize, we tell ourselves it's probably nothing. But our bodies are constantly communicating with us, and we need to listen when something feels different.

After a while, I decided to go and see what this was about, and I scheduled a doctor's appointment. They took a piece of it and sent it for a biopsy. The waiting period was agonizing. Every day felt like a week. I tried to continue my normal routine, but there was this underlying anxiety that I couldn't shake. I kept praying, but I also kept preparing myself mentally for news I didn't want to hear.

Well, the Holy Spirit prepared me. I knew that it was cancer. I just did not know why. I kept going over and over in my mind: "How could this have happened to me? I've never smoked anything a day in my life."

As it turned out, the test came back positive for cancer of the mouth/oropharynx. The official diagnosis came on May 3, 2021—a date that will forever be etched in my memory. I wasn't too shocked because the Holy Spirit had prepared me for it. I still wondered, though, *why? How?* I truly didn't understand. I said, "Me, God? But I'm your favorite."

Oddly enough, I wasn't afraid. I was confused, hurt, and questioning, but not afraid. There's a difference between fear and bewilderment, and I was definitely bewildered.

The Cascade of Challenges

This diagnosis came on the heels of what felt like a series of health challenges. I had just been diagnosed with Type 1 diabetes at 50+ years old. I had just gotten over having shingles and carpal tunnel surgery. This was just the next thing in the lineup.

I remember thinking, "Really, God? What is this about?" But even in my questioning, I knew that God was still good. Sometimes our circumstances don't reflect His goodness, immediately, but His character never changes.

On May 11, 2021, I met with my oncologist for the first time. After that appointment, I had appointment upon appointment upon appointment with oncologists, dietitians, nurses, and so forth. Each appointment brought new information, new procedures, new things to worry about. The medical world became my "new normal," and I had to learn a whole new vocabulary of terms I never wanted to know.

The Plan That Broke My Heart

They told me they could remove the lump, and after that, I would have radiation. I thought, "Okay, this isn't so bad. I can handle this."

Then they told me they would have to remove my teeth that were attached to the lump. They couldn't get the lump without removing my teeth. During the consultation, they said they would have to take some teeth. I had no idea it would be six teeth!

This hit me like a gut punch. I've been told I have a beautiful smile, and I remember a single tear falling down my face. Just one tear, but it carried the weight of a thousand fears.

My smile had always been one of my favorite features. It was how I greeted people, how I expressed joy, how I connected with others. The thought of losing that part of myself felt like losing a piece of my identity.

They also told me I would receive implants after healing. I held onto that hope like a lifeline, thinking at least my smile could eventually be restored.

"God, I don't understand, but for your glory..." I whispered through that tear.

> *"Trust in the Lord with all your heart and lean not on your own understanding; in all your ways submit to him, and he will make your paths straight."*
> **- Proverbs 3:5-6 (ESV)**

Surgery

Weeks later, on May 28, 2021, I had surgery, which went well and was considered successful. There were no complications during the procedure—something my medical team celebrated. The surgery was smooth, precise, and everything went according to plan.

The immediate aftermath of surgery was disorienting. Waking up with a different mouth, different sensations, different limitations. My husband Leroy was there, and I could see the worry in his eyes even though he tried to smile for me.

We've been married for 36 years now—I met him when I was 15 and he was 18. We have a lifetime together. I can imagine it was hard for him to see me hooked up to wires and cords, swollen from surgery and not fully conscious. He later told me he was angry that the surgery had to happen at all. He doesn't care what I look like—he loves me for me. He didn't like seeing me that way, and I can completely understand that.

I was discharged on June 3, 2021, ready to face the next phase of treatment.

The Radiation Journey

It wouldn't take long before it was time for the next thing, which was radiation. They scheduled six weeks of treatment, every weekday from July 6 through August 27, 2021. Radiation was an uncomfortable and often painful experience. I was told I could possibly lose my taste buds, my throat would be sore and raw, and I was in for a rocky road ahead.

I thought, "Nope, I'm a woman of faith. I'm believing that's not going to happen to me." My faith was high, and I refused to believe or accept the worst.

But as the radiation continued, another devastating blow came. I was told that because of the severity of the radiation, the implants I had been promised were no longer possible. Radiation had destroyed my gums too much—they couldn't support implants. Another disappointment, another adjustment to what my new normal would look like.

Instead, I would need dentures. I hate them! Even now, I'm still trying to learn how to talk without it being obvious that I have a foreign object in my mouth.

I remember three weeks into radiation, I was sitting down to a meal with my family at a restaurant and couldn't taste what I was eating. The food was there, I could see it, I could feel the texture, but the flavors that should have brought joy and satisfaction were completely gone.

And so, it began.

After a few more weeks, my throat became raw. I had sores in my throat, and I couldn't swallow. Simple acts like drinking water became challenges. Eating became a struggle. My family watched helplessly as I tried to navigate these basic human needs.

Then, nearing the end of radiation treatment, I lost my voice completely.

The silence was deafening.

I am a social person. I love my friends and family. I love conversing with them, and suddenly I couldn't verbally converse with them. I couldn't sing, and I love to sing. I couldn't speak words of encouragement to others, which had always been part of my calling.

Although my body was under attack, my spirit continuously said, "to God be the glory," while my heart was hurting. This was the hardest part—maintaining my faith declarations while feeling like I was losing pieces of myself daily.

Initially, when my voice began to return about a month and a half later, I sounded like I had a potato in my mouth. It sounded like that because I didn't have any teeth where the surgery had been. I laugh about it now, but I was very self-conscious about it then.

Family Love in the Midst of Loss

My family was wonderful during this time. Of course, they were concerned, but we are a praying, Bible-believing family. Even when sad news comes, we trust God. My husband and kids were honestly scared but very supportive. They're amazing.

My oldest daughter, Lorissa, said something that still gives me chills: "Mommy, I see angels in the room." She encouraged me and said, "You're going to be fine, and when you recover, you'll be better than you were before."

Children often see what adults miss. Her words weren't just encouragement, they were prophecy. Don't be so quick to dismiss your children's words.

I remember my girls Leydi and Leticia were planning a trip and wanted to cancel it because they didn't want to leave me. I told them, "You better go, I'll be here when you get back." They prepared meals for me and prayed for me. They even had their friends praying for me. They fixed me food, made shakes, and went to doctor's appointments with me.

This is what family does—they hold you up when you can't hold yourself up. They speak for you when you have no voice. They believe for you when your faith feels weak.

Leroy made shakes and soup for me because that's all I could tolerate. He learned to communicate with me through gestures and written notes. He became my voice when I needed to communicate with others. This man who married me for better or worse was proving what "worse" really meant, and he was choosing "better" every day. Even now they tell me that I'm beautiful even though I don't feel attractive. I'm trying to be positive for them.

Finding Voice in Voicelessness

I sat with women in the waiting room who were also waiting for radiation and some of them chemotherapy. I prayed with them, encouraged them, and I lifted them up, while my heart was breaking.

Even without my voice, I found ways to minister. I would write notes of encouragement. I would hold hands and pray silently. I would smile—even though it looked different than before—and let my eyes speak love and hope.

I thought I was being punished, but I know God doesn't do that. Going through this can cause confusion and frustration. I just kept repeating, like a mantra, "This is all for His glory."

But honestly, there were days when that felt more like something I was *supposed* to say rather than something I truly felt. Faith doesn't mean you never question or struggle, it means you keep holding on even when you don't understand.

The Long Wait for Restoration

I thought after three months, which in my mind was a reasonable amount of time, my singing voice would return. It did not.

I waited a year; it did not return.

After two years, I was able to speak better, but I could not sing.

My singing voice did not return until 2½ years later.

Do you know how long 2½ years feels when the thing you're waiting for is connected to your identity and calling? It feels like a lifetime. It feels like God has forgotten you. It feels like maybe this is just how things will be forever.

Learning to speak again was humbling. Every conversation was a reminder of what I had lost. Every attempt at singing was a reminder of what I was still waiting to regain.

But slowly, gradually, my voice began to return. Not the same voice I had before, but a new voice. A voice that had been through fire and come out refined.

> *"But he knows the way that I take;*
> *when he has tested me, I will come forth as gold."*
> **- Job 23:10 (ESV)**

During this journey, someone asked me, "What if God doesn't want you to sing? Will you be okay with that?"

I wrestled with that question. I cried and prayed and cried some more. I'm not a professional singer by any means. I never had a desire for that. What I wanted was to be used by God. Whether that was through song, teaching the Word of God, prayer, edifying, counseling, or speaking a word of prophecy, that's all I've ever wanted.

My desire has always been that God be with me and use me for His glory.

But here's what I realized: I had counted myself out after being diagnosed with oral cancer. All the aforementioned things require me to have a voice, and I thought without my original voice, I was useless to God.

Through this journey, God reminded me I am who He says I am, not who my circumstances say I am.

I had always trusted God, but this time it was something different. I had to let go of what I thought should happen and allow God to do it His way. I had to surrender not just my voice, but my expectations, my timeline, and my understanding of how God works.

The hardest part was losing my voice because I love to sing, but I have recently come to terms with the fact that it probably won't ever be the same. That fact is painful, at times. I don't like what I look like. I just see the scars from having had cancer while not knowing how it happened. I am, however, grateful to have my life.

"Be anxious for nothing, but in everything by prayer and supplication, with thanksgiving, let your requests be made known to God."
- Philippians 4:6 (ESV)

The title of my chapter is "Voice on the Altar" because that's exactly what this journey required—placing my voice, my identity, my calling, and my expectations on God's altar.

An altar is a place of sacrifice, but it's also a place of transformation. What goes on the altar doesn't always die—sometimes it's refined, purified, and given back in a new form.

I thank God that I have more to offer Him than my voice. I discovered that worship isn't just a song, it's a surrendered will. It's a heart that surrenders to God's way, even if it's not what you wanted or thought it would be.

During those 2½ years of silence and recovery, I learned to worship in new ways. I worshipped through my patience. I worshipped through my trust during the unknown. I worshipped through my acceptance of a new normal.

Life After the Test

It wasn't until after 2½ years that I was able to sing something. The first time I sang again, I cried. Not just because I could sing, but because I understood that God had given me something better than my old voice—He had given me a testimony.

Today, I'm able to sing "To God be the glory," and it means more now than it ever did before. It's because of Him that I am who I am. It's because of God that I live and breathe and have my being. It's because of Him that I am here today.

> *"For in him we live and move and have our being."*
> **- Acts 17:28 (ESV)**

My voice sounds different now. My smile looks different. My approach to ministry has evolved. But my heart for God has only grown stronger.

I've learned that God doesn't just restore—He renews. He doesn't just give back what was taken—He gives something better suited for the new season He's preparing you for.

Daily life looks different now. I have to be more intentional about dental care and oral health. I have to think about what I eat and how I eat it. Social situations sometimes require explanation or extra grace from others.

I eat whatever I want now. I remember the first time I was able to bite a sandwich after treatment—it's the little things. I'm such a foodie, so to be able to eat without having to break things down to smaller portions is awesome.

But I've also learned to see beauty in different places. I've learned that confidence doesn't come from perfect teeth or a perfect voice—it comes from knowing who you are in God.

My marriage grew stronger through this trial. Leroy and I learned to communicate in new ways. We learned that love really is "in sickness and in health," and that commitment means staying even when things get difficult.

My daughters learned to see their mother as more than just the woman who had always taken care of them. They learned to be caregivers, prayer warriors, and sources of strength. Our relationships deepened through shared struggle.

All of the cancer is gone. Praise God! I am truly grateful, and I am enjoying this part of my life. I have a new daughter—my son got married. We have a bonus granddaughter from that marriage and a new grandson. Life is grand.

Yes, I sometimes mourn the voice I had, but I'm looking forward to what God has to say with the one I have now.

To My Sister Walking This Path

I want to leave you with this: Trust Him. Trust the process. You may not understand why you were diagnosed with cancer, and why you have this battle, but the battle is the Lord's. Lean on Him daily.

If you're facing cancer that affects how you look, how you speak, how you eat, or how others see you, know that you are still beautifully and wonderfully made. Your worth isn't determined by what cancer takes away—it's determined by what God says about you.

If your identity has been shaken because your abilities have changed, remember that God's calling on your life isn't dependent on your physical abilities. He can use you in ways you never imagined, even with limitations you never expected.

If you're struggling with self-confidence because you look different than before, know that true beauty comes from within. People who matter will see your heart, not just your appearance.

And if you're wondering whether God is still good when hard things happen to good people, let me tell you: He is. His goodness isn't measured by our circumstances—it's proven by His faithfulness through every circumstance.

Today, I'm able to sing, "To God be the glory." Not with my old voice, but with my new one. Not with my old understanding, but with refined wisdom. Not despite what I went through, but because of how it changed me.

My voice was placed on the altar, and God gave it back transformed. The offering was accepted, the sacrifice was honored, and the restoration exceeded what I lost.

Whatever you're being asked to place on God's altar today—your appearance, your abilities, your expectations, your timeline—know that He can be trusted with it. What goes on the altar in surrender comes back as testimony.

"And we know that in all things God works for the good of those who love him, who have been called according to his purpose."
- Romans 8:28 (ESV)

Sing your new song, sister. The world needs to hear it.

Dear Sister,

I pray that my chapter, "The Bald Eagle" will inspire you to know that God will not leave or forsake you during this Cancer Journey. Bald Eagles have been adored for centuries as symbols of **Strength, Freedom, Power, and Spiritual Connection.** Know as you travel through this cancer journey and look unto the hills from whence cometh your help that the Lord will guide and direct you through this Wilderness Experience. I pray that you too will gain the Courage/ Strength, Divine Wisdom and Freedom that I have received through this Cancer Journey.

And please know that I am here to support you. I truly embrace the concept of meeting a person where they are, and I look forward to partnering with you. If you have questions and concerns, I would be honored to help you to explore/find the information you need.

Marisa

The Bald Eagle
"Bald and Beautiful"

Authored By: Marisa Youngblood

For centuries, bald eagles have been revered as symbols of strength, freedom, power, and spiritual connection. According to Native American beliefs, bald eagles are considered sacred and believed to act as messengers between humans and the Creator.

The bald eagle is a large, powerful bird that has been the national symbol of the United States since 1782 when it was first placed with outspread wings on the country's Great Seal as a sign of strength. My cancer journey—not one battle, but two—reminds me of the bald eagle, giving me strength, courage, divine wisdom, and freedom.

Like the eagle that soars through storms and emerges stronger, I have learned to navigate the wilderness of cancer with wings that have been tested by fire but not broken by trial.

> *"But they that wait upon the Lord shall renew their strength; they shall mount up with wings as eagles; they shall run, and not be weary; and they shall walk, and not faint."*
> **Isaiah 40:31 (KJV)**

Strength and Courage: The First Flight

January 21, 2020, is a day I will never forget. To God be the glory! I don't look like what I've been through.

I genuinely believed I would receive good news that day. "Your results were negative for breast cancer." After all, my routine mammogram in May 2019 had come back clear. But I couldn't have been more wrong.

Two days before January 21, 2020, I had just returned from out of state after dealing with a family crisis, and the very next day, a close girlfriend passed away from pancreatic cancer. I was already devastated by everything that was happening, so I convinced myself that I would be getting good news from the Cancer Center.

I was so sure of it that I asked my husband to come with me to the appointment so we could celebrate what I believed would be positive results. I also wanted to celebrate the incredible Ancestry DNA discovery of a biological sister—life seemed to be giving me gifts, so surely this appointment would be another one.

However, at 11:15 a.m., all of that changed.

As the Nurse Navigator walked in, I could tell by the look on her face that the news was not good. She explained that she had both some bad and good news. I had Invasive Ductal Carcinoma Cancer in my right breast. She explained that the good news was that it was curable.

What a relief! Through the tears and my praises to God, I managed to schedule follow-up appointments with both the surgeon and the oncologist. As I walked out the door, I felt empowered, finally able to experience some joy. I reassured my husband that he did not need to accompany me to the follow-up appointments. Knowing the cancer was curable, I felt confident that I could handle it.

But confidence built on incomplete information is fragile, and mine was about to shatter.

When Confidence Crumbles

A week later, that joy changed dramatically when I saw the surgeon. She asked, "Why are you seeing me and not the oncologist?" She then asked if I had been informed of the additional findings.

Teary-eyed and choked up, I said no, I had not been told, and that my oncologist appointment was scheduled for the following week.

Now, I was confused, perplexed, and frightened by what she shared. Reportedly, the cancer in my right breast appeared too large for surgery, and the diagnostic testing identified the tumor as being HER2+ and possibly being "Metastatic." I had no clue what any of this meant, and her bedside manner was horrible.

She said the oncologist would discuss the course of treatment and that I would probably need the following scans: lung, liver, bone, and brain to determine if the cancer had spread to those areas. I was also informed that the insurance company would have to be contacted to decide if I was a suitable candidate for surgery.

She suggested that once I calmed down, I should research HER2+ and Metastatic.

The clinical coldness of her delivery felt like a second diagnosis. Not only did I have cancer, but I was receiving this life-altering information from someone who seemed to view me as a case study rather than a human being facing her greatest fear.

Believe me, I did exactly that: research. I learned that about 15 to 20 percent of breast tumors have higher levels of a protein called HER2. Breast cancer cells with higher-than-normal levels of HER2 are classified as HER2-positive. These cancers tend to grow and spread faster than HER2-negative breast cancers, but they are also more likely to respond to targeted treatments.

I also researched metastatic breast cancer, also known as advanced or Stage Four breast cancer. This is when cancer spreads from the breast to other parts of the body. While it cannot be cured, healthcare providers can recommend treatments to improve quality of life and extend survival.

The words "cannot be cured" echoed in my mind like a death sentence.

Confronting the Past

During my weeklong wait for the oncologist appointment, I didn't know whether I would make it emotionally. Panic, fear, and anxiety knocked at my door, and I reverted to that eleven-year-old little girl who watched her mother suffer from and eventually pass away from uterine cancer.

I remember feeling helpless and not being able to help her. In class, I worried every time I heard a siren, hoping it wasn't at my house. I was scared to walk inside for fear that my mom had passed away.

On March 31, 1969, with her six children and other family members at her bedside, my mother made her heavenly transition. I couldn't understand why God had taken our forty-three-year-old mother, who was a single parent with children ranging from ages 2-16.

As angry and scared as I was, my siblings and I made it through life's ups and downs with much prayer, love, and support from our family, church family, and the community. We became productive adults with spouses, children, and grandchildren.

But now, at 62 and preparing for retirement, I was not only facing cancer but the terrifying possibility that it had already spread to my vital organs. This could not be happening.

I had always convinced myself that I would be like my mother and pass away from cancer at 43. But when I turned 44, those fears slowly faded as the years went by. At 62, I thought I had escaped that family legacy.

However, the week of waiting to see the oncologist took me back to a place I never wanted to return to. On top of that, I was still dealing with a family crisis, grieving my girlfriend's passing, and preparing to speak at her memorial, as her daughter had asked me to.

I had not yet shared my diagnosis with my daughter, son, or grandchildren. In 2019, two of my grandsons lost their father to lung cancer, and the last thing I wanted was for my family to carry the weight of worry for me. I knew it was best to wait until after my oncologist appointment and any necessary tests before telling them.

The isolation of carrying this secret felt almost as heavy as the diagnosis itself.

Finding My Wings

After much praying, fasting, and asking the Lord to give me the strength and courage to face this diagnosis, I found both through reading and meditating on God's word. The verse that carried me through was:

> *"I will lift mine eyes unto the hills, from whence cometh my help. My help cometh from the Lord, which made heaven and earth."*
> **Psalm 121:1-2 (KJV)**

Finally, the day arrived for my husband and me to meet with the oncologist and his medical team. The contrast between this doctor and the surgeon was like night and day. The oncologist was very compassionate and nurturing in his explanation of my cancer diagnosis, the stages (I-IV) of cancer, and the explanations of my next steps and phases of treatment—a two-year plan.

He drew a roadmap, explaining that my upcoming tests and scans would determine if the cancer was curable and/or treatable. We scheduled genetic testing (family history) and outpatient surgery for the chemo port, a small device that is surgically implanted under the skin to deliver chemotherapy medications directly into a vein.

I felt much better hearing his explanation of my diagnosis, course of treatment, and his validation that it was okay not to feel OK. He confirmed that the "UNKNOWN" can be the hardest part of the treatment process.

This doctor treated me like a whole person, not just a medical case, and that made all the difference in my ability to face what was ahead.

With God's help, I was able to mount up my wings like eagles, run on and not be weary, walk and not faint as I spoke at my girlfriend's memorial, shared results with my family and friends, and prepared myself for the treatment process.

Divine Wisdom: Learning to Soar

> *"Blessed is the man that trusteth in the Lord, and whose hope the Lord is."*
> **Jeremiah 17:7 (KJV)**

After a couple of weeks of sleepless nights, I prayed, fasted, and asked the Lord to give me Divine Wisdom in handling all that I was going through. To God be the glory for answering my prayers. A series of tests and scans revealed that the cancer had not spread beyond my lymph nodes.

The relief was overwhelming. What we had feared might be Stage IV metastatic cancer was actually contained. I could breathe again.

On February 20, 2020, my two-year active treatment plan and ten-year maintenance began.

My husband faithfully accompanied me to chemo treatments for the first four weeks. By March 2020, the COVID-19 pandemic was rampant, but my faith and love for the Lord grew stronger. The world was shutting down just as I was beginning the fight for my life.

Treatment Thursdays (4-6 hours) became Study and Meditation Time with God, receiving His divine wisdom. With the world in lockdown, I had no choice but to face this journey with fewer distractions and more focus on what truly mattered.

My daughter, son, grandchildren, family, friends, church family, co-workers, therapist, and groups such as "Taking Our Lives Back" were a phenomenal support. I also received many care packages, resources, and excellent books. However, two books that are dear and near to my heart are "Prayers for Difficult Times and Cancer" and "Navigating Your Cancer Journey - Handbook for Cancer Patients and Caregivers by Oncology Nurse Navigator."

Both books provided me with divine wisdom and got me through some tough times; they are excellent examples of Romans 8:26: "Likewise, the Spirit also helpeth our infirmities: for we know not what we should pray for as we ought: but the Spirit itself maketh intercession for us with groanings which cannot be uttered."

The Physical Battle

I certainly had some tough times and did not know what to pray for as my body was burned inside and out, fingernails and toenails lifting, blood vessels breaking in my eyes, sores inside my mouth and nose, removal of a portion of my right breast and lymph nodes through the lumpectomy surgical procedure and losing hair from all parts of my body, especially my head, eventually becoming:

BALD & BEAUTIFUL

The physical assault on my body was unlike anything I had ever experienced. Each day brought new challenges, new side effects, new reminders that poison was coursing through my veins to save my life. The irony was not lost on me—I had to nearly die to live.

With the world shut down, I could not work, attend church services, participate in community events, travel, or visit with family and friends. All I could do was seek God's divine wisdom and guidance.

Zoom became a lifesaver, allowing me to continue seeking divine wisdom by attending church services and weekly Bible study, visiting family and friends, attending weekly counseling and therapy sessions, and participating in a variety of activities: drumming, chair yoga, meditation through the Cancer Center, and walking 5,000 steps when my body allowed.

The isolation of COVID combined with the isolation of cancer treatment created a unique kind of wilderness experience, but it was in this wilderness that I learned to truly depend on God's provision.

Victory Bells

March 22, 2021, my mammogram showed no sign of cancer, and on April 8, 2021, I completed my last targeted therapy session, feeling blessed and excited to ring the bell signifying completion of treatment for the third time (representing the Father, Son & Holy Spirit):

1. July 2020 - completing the first round of chemotherapy
2. October 2020 - completing radiation treatment
3. April 2021 - completing targeted therapy

My infusion port was removed on May 5, 2021, and I took a three-month break from any form of chemo before starting the one-year oral medication. I was grateful the Lord had healed my body as my journey continued.

July 25, 2022, I completed one year of oral chemo medication, and began taking hormone pills through March 2030. In April 2024, my oncologist informed me that my 3D mammogram looked good and that I had graduated to begin seeing the Nurse Practitioner annually.

All praises to God.

As God would have it, April 8, 2025, the Nurse Practitioner confirmed my five-year breast cancer medical clearance from HER2 Positive tumors. Research shows that Black women have lower survival rates from this type of cancer than any other racial or ethnic group. Receiving this clearance was cause for praising and thanking God that I had made it this far.

I thought I was free. I thought my cancer journey was behind me. I thought I could finally exhale completely.

But sometimes God's plans for our testimony require more chapters than we anticipated.

The Second Storm

Listen y'all, April 16, 2025, began a different cancer journey.

I saw an endocrinologist for diabetes management. During this routine visit, she discovered nodules in my thyroid. In the following weeks, I underwent multiple ultrasounds, scans, blood tests, and biopsies. Praise God, the biopsy showed the nodules in my thyroid were benign.

But life has a way of taking unexpected turns. Satan thought he had me for sure... but GOD.

During the time of thyroid testing, I ended up in the Emergency Room for difficulty swallowing. Additional exams and X-rays yielded negative results and a referral to a gastroenterologist. Praise God for divine intervention—the gastroenterologist completed a scope and reviewed bloodwork from previous labs, discovering that my liver enzyme panel was extremely high. A panel retest showed even higher results.

The gastroenterologist recommended that I follow up with my oncologist.

After weeks of tests, I was diagnosed with Hepatocellular Carcinoma (liver cancer), identified as a secondary cancer unrelated to breast cancer and without metastasis.

I was shocked. How could this be? I was having no symptoms other than weight loss, and I didn't pay any attention to that because I'm an avid walker—10,000+ steps per day. The physicians inquired about my medical history, including any previous alcohol consumption and diagnoses of conditions such as hepatitis. The answer was no, no, no.

Here I was, five years cancer-free from breast cancer, only to face an entirely different cancer. The emotional whiplash was overwhelming. Just when I thought I could finally live without the specter of cancer hanging over my head, I was thrust back into that familiar yet unwelcome world of oncology appointments, treatment plans, and uncertainty.

The Second Flight

But this time felt different. I wasn't the same woman who had received her first cancer diagnosis in 2020. This time, I had experience. I had already learned to spread my wings during a storm. I had already discovered that my faith could carry me through the wilderness.

The cancer was detected at an early stage, and a liver resection was performed on June 17, 2025. Praise God, they were able to remove that portion of my liver, and no additional treatment was needed. However, I will have scans and bloodwork every 90 days.

The recovery from liver surgery was different from my breast cancer treatment. Instead of the prolonged assault of chemotherapy, this was a surgical strike—swift, precise, and hopefully definitive. But the emotional processing was more complex because I was dealing with the reality of being a two-time cancer survivor.

Fast-forwarding to September 2025, I know the Lord is not finished with me and continues to speak to my heart as He uses me to educate, support, and witness to others.

Freedom: Soaring with Purpose

"And to the woman were given two wings of a great eagle, that she might fly into the wilderness, into her place, where she is nourished for a time, and times, and half a time, from the face of the serpent."
Revelation 12:14 (KJV)

These experiences with cancer continue to reinforce the importance of embracing freedom. The Oxford Dictionary states that freedom is the power or right to act, speak, or think as one wants without hindrance or restraint.

But my understanding of freedom has deepened through facing cancer twice. True freedom isn't the absence of trials—it's the ability to soar through them with purpose and grace.

I have the freedom and understanding to:

Spend more time with God, seeking courage, strength, and His divine wisdom. Cancer has taught me that time with God isn't a luxury—it's essential fuel for the journey.

Exhibit Agape Love to my family and friends. Facing mortality twice has shown me that love is the only currency that truly matters.

Make healthy choices as they relate to diet, exercise, and relaxation. My body has been through so much, and I honor it by caring for it well.

Volunteer as peer support and educate others going through cancer treatment. My dual diagnosis has given me unique insight into different types of cancer journeys.

Participate in various African American cancer research projects. Representation in research matters, especially given the survival disparities I've personally overcome.

Fundraise for various cancer initiatives. Having benefited from research and support, I feel called to give back.

Participate in cancer support groups and classes. Community has been essential to my survival, and I want to provide that for others.

Communicate my health needs to both my medical and mental health professionals. I've learned to be my own advocate and to speak up when something doesn't feel right.

The Eagle's Testimony

Today, I stand as a two-time cancer survivor, bald and beautiful, with wings that have been tested by two different storms but have not been broken. Like the bald eagle that can soar at heights of 10,000 feet and see prey from miles away, cancer has given me perspective and vision I wouldn't have otherwise.

My hair has grown back—twice. My strength has returned—twice. My faith has been tested—twice—and has proven faithful both times.

I don't know if there will be a third cancer journey. I don't know what the future holds. But I know Who holds the future, and I know that whatever comes, He will give me wings to soar above it.

The eagle doesn't avoid the storm—it uses the storm's winds to rise higher. That's what I've learned to do with cancer. Each diagnosis, each treatment, each moment of uncertainty has become wind beneath my wings, lifting me to heights of faith and purpose I never knew were possible.

Closing Prayer and Praise

Thank You, Lord, for giving me two wings of a great eagle and nourishing me to withstand not one but two wilderness experiences. Thank You for the courage, strength, divine wisdom, and freedom that I have received.

I'm thankful for being healed twice, allowing me to keep serving. I appreciate my supportive community: husband, children, family, church, friends, colleagues, and others who stood by me through both challenges.

Thank You for proving that what the enemy meant for evil, You have turned for good. Thank You for showing me that being "bald and beautiful" isn't just about losing hair to chemotherapy—it's about being stripped down to what truly matters and finding beauty in survival, strength in struggle, and purpose in pain.

Continue to lift me in prayer as I continue this journey in life. To anyone facing the challenges of cancer—whether for the first time or facing recurrence—know that in Jesus' precious name, through His grace and mercy, we can all be survivors!

The eagle soars not because the storm has passed, but because she has learned to use the storm to rise higher.

Amen, Amen, Amen.
Bald and Beautiful.

"He gives strength to the weary and increases the power of the weak. Even youths grow tired and weary, and young men stumble and fall; but those who hope in the Lord will renew their strength. They will soar on wings like eagles; they will run and not grow weary, they will walk and not be faint."
Isaiah 40:29-31 (ESV)

Dear Sister,

I didn't know what was going to happen, but all of this has taught me to live for today, not tomorrow. (Matthew 6:34) I want to live my life for God, even though it's a struggle. But hey, it's one day at a time. I'm choosing myself for a change because tomorrow isn't promised. I want you to remember to keep praying, put God first, and always maintain a positive attitude, no matter what.

                                                  Monica

My Journey Ain't Yours, and Yours Isn't Mine

Authored By: Monica Poe

I'm not good with feelings. Never have been. People always want me to explain how something "made me feel" or what was "going through my mind" when this or that happened. Truth is, I don't always know. I'm more of an "it is what it is" kind of person. Always have been. Some folks call it being strong. Others say I'm in denial. But that's just who I am—I deal with what's in front of me and keep moving.

Problem is, when you're a 46-year-old Black woman who's been through what I've been through, people expect you to have more words for it all. They expect tears and breakdowns and deep spiritual revelations. And maybe I should. Maybe there's something wrong with me that I don't. But I'm gonna tell you my story the way I know how to tell it—straight, no chaser, and with the understanding that some things just don't fit into neat little emotional packages.

I'm a mom, wife, and only child. Life has been challenging from the start—one thing after another. But that's not a complaint; that's just facts. My childhood was okay, but I had to grow up quickly, doing things I had no business doing at an early age. My mom had me when she was only 18, so needless to say, she did her best with what she knew.

Looking back now, I realize I learned early that life comes at you fast, and you either roll with it or get rolled over. I chose to roll with it.

When the Pattern Started

Fast forward to Mom's forties—she was diagnosed with breast cancer. Now, I know I'm supposed to tell you about the devastating phone call or the moment our world stopped, but honestly, I don't remember it being like that. Mom was always practical about things, and I guess I got that from her. She told me matter-of-factly, and I received it the same way.

What I do remember is the frustration. Not the crying, emotional kind of frustration, but the practical kind. Mom didn't get treatment right away. I still don't know if it was fear, denial, or just hoping it would go away, but by the time she sought help, she was at stage four.

People ask me if I was angry with her for waiting. I struggle to put that into words because anger feels too simple for what I felt. It was more like… helplessness, I guess. Like watching someone you love choose a path you can't redirect them from. But even that doesn't capture it completely. Maybe some feelings just don't have words.

Mom had her ups and downs with chemotherapy and fought a good fight, but she lost her battle at the age of 48. I was devastated—though I'm not sure that word covers it either. I also found some peace knowing she didn't have to suffer anymore. I was grateful to have had her in my life for as long as I did, and thankful that I was already an adult by the time she passed.

See, that's what I mean about feelings. People expect me to tell you about sobbing at her bedside or having some profound last conversation. But it wasn't like that. It was quiet and sad and final, and I dealt with it the way I deal with everything—by accepting it and figuring out what came next.

But I was able to tell her that I would be okay and that she did a good job. Moments later, I watched her take her last breath.

Living Under a Shadow

After Mom passed, I made it a priority to get my mammograms every year like clockwork. I wasn't being paranoid—I was being practical. Cancer runs in my family, and I knew that. My mom, my grandmother, my cousin, two aunts, and even an uncle had all battled it. Some survived, and others didn't. That's just the hand we were dealt.

For years, everything was fine. I'd go to my appointment, get the results, and move on with my life. I didn't spend time worrying about what might happen because, honestly, what's the point? Either it happens or it doesn't, and worrying won't change that.

But somewhere in the back of my mind, I always knew this day might come. Not in a fearful way, just in a realistic way. Like knowing you might get caught in traffic or that it might rain. You don't plan your whole life around it, but you're not completely surprised when it happens.

At 44, I was diagnosed with stage two breast cancer.

I'll never forget when my doctor called to give me the news, though probably not for the reasons you'd think. I was at the store, and she asked if she could call me back when I got home. That alone let me know it wasn't good news. But when she finally told me, I remained calm. I didn't cry, and I didn't feel any fear.

People always want to know what I was thinking in that moment. Truth is, I was thinking about practical things. Who I needed to call. What I needed to do next. How to tell my family. That's just how my brain works—straight to the logistics.

I know I'm supposed to tell you about being scared or angry or having some spiritual crisis, but that's not what happened. Cancer wasn't new to me. It had been circling my family for years like some unwelcome relative who shows up uninvited but you can't quite get rid of. In some weird way, I'd been preparing for this conversation my whole life.

During all of this, I found out that I'm BRCA2 positive, which means I carry the gene. Now that hit different. Not for me—I was already dealing with my situation. But for my daughter. Because of this, she'll need to start getting checked as early as 18 years old.

That's the part that's hard to put into words. How do you tell your child she inherited something from you that could kill her? How do you wrap your mind around passing down a legacy of potential death instead of just your eyes or your laugh? I struggle with that one because there aren't easy answers, and "it is what it is" doesn't quite cover it.

The Battle I Never Signed Up For

I began chemotherapy on February 14th, 2022. Valentine's Day. If that ain't irony, I don't know what is. Treatment lasted until June 2022, and let me tell you, it felt like it went on forever.

One of the treatments I had was called the "Red Devil." Now, I'd heard some terrifying stories about this one, but thankfully, my experience was different. Maybe it's because I don't fight against things I can't control, maybe I just got lucky, or maybe the Lord knows that I can't handle all of that, and had mercy on me. Either way, I rolled with it.

The main challenges I faced were losing my hair, losing my taste buds (which didn't come back for a whole year), and numbness in my hands and feet, which I still deal with, though it's not as bad as it was. I didn't lose weight or get sick, and I was able to keep up with most of my usual activities, aside from feeling more tired during the day.

When it came to my hair, I remember having a headache that lasted three days. It felt like my hair was trying to come out from the root, so I asked my husband to cut it all off. As soon as he did, the headaches stopped. Simple as that.

People want to know if I mourned my hair or felt less feminine or had some emotional breakdown about it. I didn't. Hair grows back. It's temporary. My body is temporary. I've got bigger things to worry about than how I look in a mirror.

This all happened during the pandemic, which added another layer of difficulty. But through it all, I just kept moving forward. That's what I do. That's what I've always done.

I didn't know what was going to happen, but all of this has taught me to live for today, not tomorrow. I want to live my life for God, even though it's a struggle. But hey, it's one day at a time.

"Therefore do not worry about tomorrow, for tomorrow will worry about itself. Each day has enough trouble of its own."
Matthew 6:34 (ESV)

The Numbers Game

Here's something I share as often as possible to encourage others God is real. In my lifetime, I've had 26 miscarriages.

Twenty. Six.

People always gasp when I tell them that number, and I understand why. It sounds impossible. It sounds devastating. It sounds like something that should have broken me completely.

But see, this is where my whole "it is what it is" thing gets complicated. Because I know I'm supposed to tell you about the grief and the loss and the dreams that died with each pregnancy. And maybe I felt those things. Maybe I should have felt them more. But what I remember most is just... moving forward. Getting up. Trying again.

Maybe that's not normal. Maybe there's something wrong with me that I can't tap into whatever other women feel when they lose pregnancies. Or maybe that's just how I survived it. I don't know. What I do know is that despite all those losses, I now have three healthy children. I had my first at 35 and my last at 40. I had them all by C-section, and when I tell you, I had no pain and was able to walk the same day.

God works in mysterious ways, and I don't pretend to understand His plan. But I know that my babies—the ones I get to hold—are miracles. Every single day with them is a gift I almost didn't get.

I've also had a double mastectomy and a full hysterectomy. People ask if I feel less like a woman or if I struggle with my identity. I struggle to answer that because I don't really know what it means to feel "less like a woman." I feel like me. Maybe different, but still me.

The Aftermath Nobody Talks About

After the chemo, my body had a reaction to one of the treatments, so I have these cheetah-type spots all over my body. When I tell people about this, they expect me to be upset or self-conscious. But this is the way I look at it: My body is a temporary body, and God has the final say in my life.

We get one life to live, so I rock my spots like I was born with them. It is not my focus. I don't care what people say or think.

But here's what I struggle to articulate—this whole experience has changed something in me that I can't quite name. Not in a dramatic, life-altering revelation kind of way, but in a quieter way. I find myself thinking about things differently. Time feels different. Priorities feel different.

I've been with the same man for 33 years. We've been married 17 years, so y'all gotta know that was nothing but God, and that's a whole book in itself. But cancer changes your relationship too, in ways nobody prepares you for. Not bad ways, necessarily, just... different ways.

He had to watch me go through treatment. He had to cut my hair when it hurt too much to keep. He had to learn to live with the uncertainty too. People focus on the patient, but the people who love us? They're fighting their own battles. Needless to say, I beat cancer, but my marriage didn't survive, and I'm still processing that. That's another book.

The Fear I Can't Shake

There aren't many things in this world that surprise me, but one thing that keeps crossing my mind is age 48. Being an only child, and with my mom passing at that age, it's a scary thought.

Now, before you get worried about me, let me be clear—I'm not planning on dying at 48. I'm not putting that energy out there or speaking that over my life. But I'd be lying if I said the thought doesn't cross my mind sometimes.

I don't know what that age will bring for me. If that means that's what's going to happen to me, then I don't have long. But I have to keep reminding myself that my mom's story isn't my story, and that may not be God's plan for me.

This is one of those things I struggle to put into words because it's not exactly fear, but it's not exactly peace either. It's like living with a question mark hanging over your head. And for someone who likes things straightforward, question marks are uncomfortable.

I also know there's power in the words you speak, so I try to be mindful of what I say. Again, that's a job in itself. The devil is always listening.

But here's what I've learned about survivorship—it's not just about surviving the cancer. It's about surviving the after. The wondering. The "what ifs." The way people look at you differently, like you're fragile when you don't feel fragile. The way every ache or pain makes you wonder if it's back.

I'm still learning how to live with that uncertainty, and some days are better than others. Some days I forget I ever had cancer. Other days, the numbness in my hands reminds me. The spots on my skin remind me. The scheduled check-ups remind me. The sporadic sharp pains in my chest remind me.

What I'm Learning About Surviving Survivorship

People think surviving cancer is about getting through treatment and ringing the bell and moving on. But survivorship is its own thing, and it's harder in some ways because there's no clear protocol for it. There's no schedule. There's no "do this for six months and you'll be fine."

Survivorship is learning to live with the knowledge that your body betrayed you once and could do it again. It's learning to make plans while holding them loosely because you know how quickly everything can change.

It's also learning that some people will treat you like you're inspirational when you don't feel inspirational. You feel normal. Like the same person who just happened to have cancer for a while.

And for someone like me—someone who doesn't naturally process emotions deeply—survivorship is confusing because everyone expects you to have learned some profound life lesson or found some deep spiritual meaning. Maybe I have and I just can't articulate it. Or maybe my lesson is simpler: that life keeps coming at you, and you keep dealing with it, and sometimes that's enough.

I'm choosing myself for a change because tomorrow isn't promised. Not in a selfish way, but in a realistic way. I want to do things I enjoy. I want to rest when I need to. I want to stop saying yes to things that don't serve me or my family.

That might not sound like a big revelation, but for someone who's spent her whole life just going with the flow and dealing with whatever comes, choosing to prioritize my own needs feels revolutionary.

Living in the Space Between

God is so worthy to be praised at all times and in all situations. See, the fact is, once you're born, you start to die. There's no way around your exit, but while you're here, just enjoy your life and keep God first, or at least do your best.

I've realized that I'm living in the space between—between sick and healthy, between past and future, between knowing and not knowing.

And maybe that's where faith lives too. In the space between certainty and uncertainty.

> *"I can do all things through Christ who strengthens me."*
> **Philippians 4:13 (ESV)**

"No temptation has overtaken you except what is common to mankind. And God is faithful; he will not let you be tempted beyond what you can bear. But when you are tempted, he will provide a way out so that you can endure it." 1 Corinthians 10:13 (ESV)

These verses remind me to trust in God's faithfulness, knowing that He is with me every step of the way, giving me the strength to endure and overcome.

To My Sisters in This Fight

If you're reading this and you've just been diagnosed, or you're in treatment, or you're learning how to be a survivor, I want you to know that there's no right way to do this. There's no right way to feel. There's no timeline for processing it all.

Maybe you're like me and you don't cry much or have dramatic spiritual awakenings. That's okay. Maybe you do, and that's okay too. Your journey ain't mine, and mine ain't yours.

What I know is this: Hold on to the Lord's unchanging hand. I know the diagnosis is scary. But we serve a good God, and He has a plan for your life. Take care of yourself. Rest when you need to, and do things in life that you enjoy. Live your life to the fullest.

And if you struggle to find words for what you're going through, that's okay too. Some experiences are bigger than words. Some feelings don't fit into neat categories. Sometimes "it is what it is" is enough, and sometimes it's not, and both can be true at the same time.

What matters is that you keep going. Keep showing up. Keep trusting that God's got you, even when you can't see the plan.

Because at the end of the day, survival isn't about having all the right feelings or saying all the right words. It's about being here tomorrow, and the day after that, and the day after that.

And that's something I know how to do.

"He heals the brokenhearted and binds up their wounds."
Psalm 147:3 (ESV)

Live your life to the fullest.
That's my prayer for you and for me.

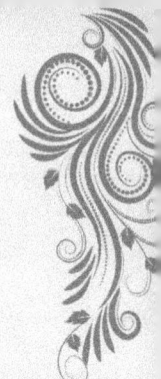

How do you see your cancer journey contributing to the broader narrative of Black women's health and resilience?

I feel that historically, black people have a background of a praying/church community. Grandma prays, Momma prays, pastor/church prays. My kids had their friends praying for me. I was covered on all ends of the spectrum.

Lisa

Dear Sister,

I pray you are encouraged by my journey. As I write, I am a 20-year cancer survivor. I hate cancer and what it does to our bodies and our lives, but at the same time, we often get to start over with a new lease on life after battling this disease. Stay hopeful.

Neicy

Fought and Won!

Authored by: Neicy Johnson

I was just driving back to work after lunch, one hand on the steering wheel, the other resting on my neck like I always did. It was February 2004, and I was 36 years old with two kids and a full life ahead of me. I had no idea that this ordinary Tuesday would be the day everything changed.

My fingers felt something that shouldn't have been there—a knot on the left side of my neck. I immediately checked the other side. Nothing. Just smooth skin where there should have been symmetry.

When I got back to work, I asked a few coworkers to feel what I was feeling. They confirmed it—there was definitely something there. But I went on about my day and thought nothing else about it. Looking back, I think part of me knew that knot was going to change my life, but I wasn't ready to face that possibility yet.

A week later, while at the hair salon, everything came crashing down. I became ill and felt like I was going to pass out. As I sat in the chair, my head was spinning, and the room went dark. That day, I decided I couldn't ignore what was happening anymore. I had to see a doctor.

I went to the emergency room the next day, and I was a nervous wreck because I had never experienced anything like that before. When I described my symptoms to the ER doctor—the dizziness and the knot—they performed a scan of my neck and my head. I was there for hours, feeling anxious about the head scan, thinking it might be a tumor or something worse.

When the doctor and nurse came in with the results, I paid attention to the look on their faces, and it wasn't what I wanted to see. The doctor, with a serious tone, said the head scan was clear, but the radiologist saw a mass in my neck and my back.

A mass? I was confused, and I knew this wasn't good. I was referred to an oncologist and scheduled for a neck biopsy.

The Waiting Game

A couple of weeks passed before the results were due to come back. During that time, I was a basket case. I tried to go on with my days as normal and not worry, but it was very difficult. Every night when I put my 13-year-old and 5-year-old to bed, I wondered if I would be there to see them grow up. Every morning when I looked in the mirror, I touched that knot and wondered what it was doing to my body.

My appointment date arrived to get my results, and I went in there prayed up, knowing that God had my back. But as I sat in that waiting room, I felt anything but confident.

As I waited for the doctor to come in with my results, I began reading one of the health magazines. There was a story about a young woman who was diagnosed with cancer. As I began reading her story, my heart began to pound with nervousness because she was me. Everything she described was exactly what I had experienced—the knot, the dizziness, the fear. I was thinking, no, I can't have cancer. I wished I had kept that magazine because I wanted to finish reading her story, to see how it ended.

But I never got the chance.

March 4, 2004: The Day Life Stopped

The doctor came into the room, and on March 4, 2004, my life changed forever. I was diagnosed with Hodgkin's Lymphoma, which is cancer of the lymph tissues. I knew nothing about it, except that it was cancer, and cancer meant death in my mind.

Of course, I was in shock. I remember the doctor saying to me, "If you have to have any type of cancer, THIS is the one you want to have because the survival rate is very high." That didn't make me feel better at all. All I heard was "cancer," and all I could think about was dying.

I've been very independent throughout my adult life, and I had handled this appointment alone because I didn't want to alarm my family. I should not have gone to that doctor by myself that day. I was crying in the office, and the nurse allowed me to sit for as long as I needed. All I could think about were my children, who were 13 and 5 years old at the time. The thought of death became my constant companion from that moment on. I was numb.

I remember the walk from the doctor's office to the car. It seemed like it took me forever to get to my car. Every step felt heavy, like I was walking through quicksand. I sat in the car and cried—deep, body-shaking sobs that came from a place I didn't know existed.

Then I called my family and friends to tell them about my diagnosis. Each phone call was harder than the last. Hearing myself say the words "I have cancer" made it more real, more terrifying.

I went home, and everything started from there. I didn't know what the outcome was going to be, but I was ready to get the ball rolling. I researched that particular cancer to get a better understanding, to be an advocate for my own health, and to know what was coming next.

After numerous tests, the results revealed the cancer was stage 3B and had spread to my neck, under both arms, my lungs, and my chest. When I heard "stage 3B," I thought I was going to die. I had not thought of living at that point. My mind went straight to funeral planning and who would take care of my babies.

"Even though I walk through the valley of the shadow of death, I will fear no evil, for you are with me; your rod and your staff, they comfort me."
Psalm 23:4 (ESV)

The Battle Begins

March 22, 2004, was the day of my first chemotherapy. When I walked into the chemo room, it was cold and dreary. The smell in the room made me want to vomit, and seeing all the people hooked up to IVs was the worst sight I could imagine. The nurse took me to my chair, made sure I was comfortable, and began hooking me up to an IV. My first chemo treatment was administered, and my treatments were scheduled for every other Monday.

My mom took care of me and helped me with my children during this time, and I am so grateful for her. Without her, I don't know how I would have managed.

It took me a minute to come to grips with it all. I was in disbelief and could not believe that I had cancer. A few months after I started chemotherapy, there were days I wanted to give up. I was tired—tired in a way I had never experienced before. The chemotherapy was rough. It made me sick, weak, and it took a toll on my body and my mind.

I cried every time I looked at the scars on my body that looked like Freddy Krueger had gotten hold of me. I struggled through days of not being able to taste my food, the nausea, fatigue, and having to deal with the pain from the sores in my mouth. I was told to avoid the sun because of one of the medications. Before I received a Medi-Port, the chemo was administered through my veins in my arm, and many days I sat there for 4 to 5 hours crying, watching the medicine slowly go into my body.

When Hope Almost Died

In May 2004, I lost two cousins that I was very close to. They both died of cancer two weeks apart, and I was a basket case. I just knew that I was next. I knew that my family would be planning my funeral next, which sent me into a deep depression that I had never experienced before.

I started questioning everything. Why was I fighting so hard if I was just going to die anyway? What was the point of putting my body through this torture if the outcome was going to be the same as my cousins'?

July 2004 was the time I wanted to end it all. I did not want to go to treatment, and I was severely depressed that day. As I was getting my chemo, I began to rip the tape from around my Medi-Port so that I could remove the needle and go home to die. I was extremely tired, and I did not want to sit there and watch that "Red Devil," as it's called in the cancer world, go into my body.

In that moment, I felt completely alone, even though I was surrounded by nurses and other patients. I felt like I was drowning, and I couldn't see any way out of the darkness that had consumed me. The physical pain was nothing compared to the emotional and mental anguish I was experiencing.

I stopped myself before I could pull the needle out completely, and I began to cry and pray. I covered my face with the blanket so no one would see me falling apart. I knew that I needed to be here for my children and that God was not done with me yet. But knowing that and feeling it were two very different things.

The Mask I Wore

My family and friends would ask me, "Neicy, are you okay?" Some would say, "You don't look like you're going through chemo." Well, little did they know that all that strength and those smiles were fake. I did it for them so they wouldn't worry about me.

I became an expert at hiding my pain. I learned to smile when I wanted to scream, to say "I'm fine" when I was anything but fine. There were days when I felt good enough to go to work or volunteer at my son's school. I needed some sense of normalcy during that time. I even drove myself to the hospital every morning to get a shot that I needed to keep my immune system up.

But behind closed doors, I was falling apart. I would cry in the shower so my children couldn't hear me. I would have panic attacks in my car after appointments. I would lie awake at night, touching my body, checking for new lumps, wondering if the cancer was spreading.

The hardest part wasn't the physical symptoms—it was pretending to be brave when I felt like I was drowning. It was protecting everyone else from my fear while I was consumed by it.

The Turning Point

In August 2004, something shifted. I put my fears behind me and decided to fight like a champion. I pushed myself through the treatments without wanting to give up. I had many conversations with God, and I asked Him to give me the strength to surpass all the fear, panic attacks, anxiety, and depression. I had so much to live for—I had my children, my family, and friends who were all rooting for me.

I realized that dying wasn't really what I wanted. What I wanted was for the pain to stop, for the fear to go away, for my life to feel normal again. But dying wasn't the answer to any of those things.

I started focusing on what I was fighting for instead of what I was fighting against. Every treatment became one step closer to holding my children's children. Every day I survived was a victory, not just an endurance test.

The Words I Prayed For

In September 2004, I was scheduled for an appointment to get results from my scan. On my way to the hospital, I saw darkness. Everything was dark to me. I felt like I couldn't hear anything. Things were moving in slow motion. It was weird. I didn't know, going into the doctor's office, what my scan would show. I was nervous, but this time it was a different kind of nervous—hopeful nervous instead of terrified nervous.

I remembered a visit where I saw a different doctor in my regular doctor's absence, and she had said, "Ms. Johnson, because your cancer is stage 3B, the cancer will most likely come back." Of course, that had scared the hell out of me, and it always stuck with me when I went in for my checkups. But today, I was choosing to hope for something different.

When my doctor came in, he told me exactly what I had prayed for: "No More Cancer!!!"

I cried through the entire visit. They were happy tears, of course, and suddenly, the darkness that I had seen coming into the hospital was no longer surrounding me. Light was everywhere—in the doctor's smile, in the nurse's congratulations, in the relief that flooded my entire body.

I thought the results meant that I was done with the treatments, but he wanted me to have two more treatments for preventive reasons. I was tired and wanted to be done, but I knew that it was coming to an end soon.

I completed my last chemotherapy on October 25, 2004, and I was declared by God and my doctor that I was cancer-free!

Taking My Life Back

In October 2024, I celebrated 20 years being cancer-free. But the journey didn't end when the treatments stopped. In many ways, that's when the real work began.

For years after my treatment ended, I allowed my diagnosis to control my life. Every time I would get sick—a cough, itchy skin, a headache (which are a few symptoms of Hodgkin's)—I thought the cancer had returned. I was spending days touching and feeling my body for knots, just like I had done with that first one in my neck.

I knew enough was enough. I could not allow the cancer to control me or control my life. I had to take my life back from the fear, from the anxiety, from the constant worry about recurrence.

During my treatments, my finances and my living expenses had suffered tremendously. I had promised God that if He saved my life, I would be a blessing to women and their families who are battling cancer. For years, I participated in cancer walks, donated to cancer organizations, and purchased items where the proceeds were donated to cancer organizations. In my heart, I knew that wasn't enough. I wanted to do more, but I didn't know what.

One day, while surfing the internet, I saw my passion. It was a calendar of women who shared their journey while battling cancer. I knew putting together something of that magnitude was not cheap, and I did not have the finances for it, so I let it go. But that strong desire to help pressed on my heart, and eventually, I was blessed with the finances. In 2013, the first "Taking Our Lives Back" calendar was born.

The title "Taking Our Lives Back" was perfect because that's exactly what we all needed to do—take our lives back from cancer, from fear, from the identity of being a patient instead of being a whole person.

Building a Community of Survivors

I had no clue what I was doing or getting into when I began to create the first calendar, but I stepped out on faith and put the plan in motion. I used my social media platform, my family and friends, and asked around for 12 women who were survivors or currently battling to share their stories—to encourage other women who are battling cancer to keep fighting and not give up on life, despite the ongoing bouts with chemotherapy, hair loss, surgeries, radiation, tears, pain, and depression.

I found a photographer, printer, graphic designer, and the rest is history. I have since created seven calendars, including the 2023 "Taking Our Lives Back" calendar that was released in October 2022.

A portion of the proceeds from the sales was donated to organizations such as:

The Barbara Ann Karmanos Cancer Institute
Lymphoma Research Foundation
Josephine Ford Cancer Center
Cancer Awareness and Resource Network
My Sistah's Pink Journey

All of which provide cancer patients and their families with assistance for living expenses and more.

I started a Facebook group for women who are cancer survivors or currently battling. I created the group so that we could have a safe place to share our stories with one another—to become a sisterhood. We celebrate each other's success stories, cancerversaries, and support each other's businesses. We encourage new women who are added to the group to stay strong, keep fighting, and let them know there is a community of supporters, family, and friends standing with them.

The Ongoing Battle

Although I am reaching 20 years cancer-free, it's still a battle. I am constantly reminded about my journey—the scars on my body left from chemotherapy, the fear of recurrence that creeps up during routine check-ups, and the struggle with survivor's remorse.

Survivor's remorse is real, and it's something I never expected to deal with. Why did I survive when my cousins didn't? Why did my treatment work when others' didn't? Why was I spared when so many others weren't? These questions don't have easy answers, but they weigh on your heart when you're a survivor.

I am in constant prayer and ask God to continue to help me take my life back and remove the things that hold me in bondage. Because even when cancer is gone from your body, it can still live in your mind if you let it.

"For I know the plans I have for you, declares the Lord, plans for welfare and not for evil, to give you a future and a hope."
Jeremiah 29:11 (ESV)

My Mission Continues

In February 2019, I started my own nonprofit named Taking Our Lives Back of Michigan. The mission of Taking Our Lives Back of Michigan is to provide support to women and their families who are impacted by cancer. Our vision is to lift the burden from women so that they can focus on healing.

The services that we provide include:

Financial support such as rent/mortgage payments, utility payments, and medical payments paid directly to consumers (when funds are available)

Chemo tote bags, gift boxes, and baskets (which include essentials needed for chemotherapy)

Family adoption during the Christmas holiday

Every woman we help is a reminder of why I fought so hard to survive. Every calendar we create is proof that cancer doesn't have the final word in our stories. Every dollar we raise is another way to take our lives back from a disease that tries to steal everything from us.

To My Sisters in the Fight

I encourage women who are newly diagnosed to be advocates for their own health—to be sure that they understand the treatments that the doctors are suggesting. Although it may be difficult at times, it's extremely important to remain positive, even when positivity feels impossible.

Once a person is diagnosed with cancer, in some cases we relate it to death instead of life. I was guilty of this myself. But being able to keep a positive outlook and live your life to the fullest as much as possible can definitely help in the fight to beat cancer.

It's okay to have dark days. It's okay to want to give up sometimes. It's okay to cry, to be angry, to question God, to feel like you can't take another step. What's important is that you don't stay in that place. What's important is that you reach out for help when you need it.

I encourage you to connect with those who have experienced this journey to help you with yours. Don't go through this alone like I tried to do. Let people love you through this. Let people help you carry the burden.

If you are on Facebook, I'd love to have you in my free community, Taking Our Lives Back. We understand what you're going through because we've been there. We know what it feels like to hear those words "you have cancer." We know what it feels like to sit in that chemo chair. We know what it feels like to wonder if you'll see your children grow up.

But we also know what it feels like to hear "no more cancer." We know what it feels like to ring that bell. We know what it feels like to celebrate another year of survival.

"She is clothed with strength and dignity; she can laugh at the days to come." Proverbs 31:25 (ESV)

You are stronger than you know. You are braver than you feel. And you are not alone in this fight.

Fight hard. Fight with everything you have. And when you're ready, help someone else fight too.

Because that's how we take our lives back—together.

Q. How has your perspective on life and priorities shifted since your experience with cancer?

Nicole Lee: Since cancer, I have recognized that every day is a blessing, and I want to live and make the best out of the day before me. My relationship with my son and parents strengthened. Our family time and their support for me has increased so much.

Dear Sister,

I am sharing my story with you to encourage you because you matter, my sister. You are victorious and the apple of God's eye. Take a look in the mirror even right now and see yourself as the overcomer and winner you were created to be. Get up, stand up, and continue to fight the good fight of faith, standing on the word of God. You're already declared victorious over cancer.

Nicole

Walk in Miracles

Authored By: Nicole Lee

The beginning of October 2022 was the end of a year like no other and truly changed my life forever. This was my transition from resigning as a patient relations manager for seven years at Hurley Medical to beginning work in the field of mental health as a Clinical Therapist. On October 31st, I was set to begin my role as a Clinical Therapist at Easter Seals MORC while also launching my private practice, Purlife Counseling.

But God had other plans for that day.

I had been feeling a hard lump in my breast that began with sharp pains and a burning sensation. When I learned that the Genesys Hurley Cancer Institute had a free screening for breast cancer, I decided to attend. This was a blessing because my new health insurance wasn't going to be active for the next thirty days.

I arrived at the Imaging Center for my mammogram, checked in at the desk, and was taken to the room for my examination. I was warmly greeted by the friendly staff and the kind breast cancer surgeon, Dr. Suzanne Law. She was personable and took the time to explain the details of what she would be doing during the screening, which put me at ease. I also had the opportunity to meet Marsha Schmidt, the breast cancer navigator from Hurley Hospital, who provided additional guidance and support during this time.

I was led into the examination room with Dr. Law, and she began my breast examination. She found the hard mass in my right breast and swollen lymph nodes under my right arm that she wanted to test further. When I explained to Dr. Law that I had no insurance for 30 days, she stated she would assist me through this situation. The breast cancer navigator informed me about available funding to help cover the cost of a mammogram and offered to aid me in applying for Medicaid. Dr. Law then coordinated with her staff, who promptly scheduled me for a mammogram appointment within the next few days.

As I drove away from the screening, the Holy Spirit spoke to me and said, "God is faithful and He won't fail."

It was at that moment I knew I had cancer. But I also knew that God was already working on my behalf.

The Diagnosis That Couldn't Shake My Faith

Once the exams were completed, I waited for a while as the image was reviewed by the radiologist. I received a call over the phone while still at the imaging place from the radiologist stating I had breast cancer. I was then scheduled for a biopsy to get more imaging.

When I arrived home, I received a phone call from my primary care physician confirming I had breast cancer. But here's the thing—I wasn't shaken because the Holy Spirit had already prepared me. I immediately contacted my only son, Colonel, and my nurse daughter-in-love, Amber, my mother, Ada, and my father, Joe, regarding being diagnosed with breast cancer. But I let them know what the Holy Spirit spoke to me as I left the first cancer screening before being diagnosed: "God is able, and He will not fail."

I held on to my faith and wholeheartedly believed in Him. They stood with me in agreement, believing in God.

"But He was wounded for our transgressions, He was bruised for our iniquities; The chastisement for our peace was upon Him, And by His stripes we are healed." Isaiah 53:5 (KJV)

Because of God's word, we can stand in agreement with what the Holy Spirit said—God is able and He won't fail.

What a way to end October. On October 31st, I was diagnosed with cancer, but the Holy Spirit reassured me, giving me peace and strength. Remarkably, this was also the same day I was hired at Easter Seals—a new job and a new season in my life. I had no idea what a life-changing ride it would be.

Fighting on Every Front

The day of my next imaging began early at 6 AM, and I had to prepare for an hour's drive to the out-of-town location. The weather wasn't the best that morning, and I got a flat tire before getting on the highway. But I was able to overcome this obstacle by calling my dad to exchange cars and get to the imaging place on time.

When I arrived, my biopsy was completed from the cancer lump itself and lymph nodes. The next imaging appointment was scheduled for a PET scan with the breast cancer surgeon once the results were completed.

The surgeon met with me, my son Colonel, and my nurse daughter-in-love, Amber, to deliver the diagnosis: I had stage 3 Metastatic Invasive Ductal Breast Cancer. The details of the diagnosis were discussed, and I was scheduled to meet with the oncologist to further discuss the plan. The surgeon let me know the mass in my breast was too large to remove before chemo and had also metastasized to my lymph nodes.

While processing this diagnosis, I was also scheduled to begin my first day of training and computer pickup before beginning my first day at my new job at Easter Seals MORC. I met with my new boss and disclosed to her that I was diagnosed with cancer before starting my official first day, letting her know I'd have further information as things progressed.

I met with the oncologist over the next few days, bringing my son and daughter-in-love along with the nurse practitioner. The oncologist and nurse practitioner took the time to answer all our questions and discuss the cancer diagnosis in detail. They outlined the treatment plan, including the chemotherapy regimen, the potential duration of treatment, and the medications involved. They also explained what to expect over the next six months, providing clarity and guidance during this challenging time.

It was so much to comprehend at once, but I knew God was in control.

The Battle for My Hair

I discussed the cancer with my hairstylist and friend, Ericka Marshall, letting her know I wanted to keep my hair. I prayed to God saying, "If I have to go through this, can I at least keep my hair?" My hairstylist told me that her aunt Pam kept her hair through chemo through cold capping and gave me her aunt's number to discuss what it entailed.

I had heard about an option called cold capping, which helps preserve hair during chemotherapy. The oncology center provided me with a social worker, and I asked her if the cancer center provided cold capping to preserve hair during chemo. She provided me with a pamphlet from Penguin Cold Caps for further information and emailed me the financial aid application and website.

I completed the financial application, and due to not receiving a paycheck yet or knowing my hours with beginning chemo, I was approved for financial aid with Penguin Cold Capping. The items were sent via FedEx overnight.

I scheduled a Zoom meeting with my son and daughter-in-law to go over what would be required for cold capping during chemotherapy, as I would need their assistance throughout the process. The cold capping process required a timer, a temperature monitor, and bands to hold the cap in place. During the Zoom call, my son and daughter-in-law were present as I tried on the cold caps. A training session was provided by a representative from Penguin Cold Cap to guide us through the process.

The only thing I needed to purchase was a freezer to keep the caps below zero during chemotherapy. I also had to buy pounds of dry ice weekly, the day before my treatments, which cost around $100 each week at local stores like Meijer and Kroger. I reached out to inquire if they offered discounts for cancer patients purchasing dry ice to preserve their hair, but I was told they didn't provide that discount.

However, I found a dry ice company, EZ Pro Delivery, in Saginaw, Michigan, about a 35-minute drive away, that offered a discounted price of $25 for chemo patients. This was a significant savings compared to the $100 I had been spending weekly. I had a friend, Carse Franklin III, who drove to Saginaw weekly to pick up the dry ice to make sure I had it for chemo that was set once a week on Thursday for 6 months.

Carried by Prayer

Starting chemo and a new job was not easy. The job at Easter Seals required seeing clients at schools, inside homes, and evening outings within the community with the clients. But I was blessed enough to have my family praying for me.

I was surrounded by an army of prayer warriors: my son Colonel and daughter-in-love Amber Lee; my parents Ada Lee, Joseph and Dorothy Lee;

my cousin Angela Vaughn and my late Aunt Delores Vaughn; Aunt Ida Johnson and her prayer bible study group; cousin Renee Lee, cousin Deborah Simmons and the entire Lee Family; aunt Virginia and uncle Bill Thompson; aunt Betty Lamar; Pete Lee; my Pastor Alfred Harris Jr. and First Lady Cimone Harris and New Jerusalem Full Gospel Church Family; Monday Morning Glory; Pastor Veotis Jones; Elder Margie Hartman; Dr. Jeffrey and Arjeta LaValley; Jeanine Mayberry; Diane; Lawrence E. Moon; Bill Quarles.

My sister friends stood with me: Karen Smith, Lesia Moses, Ketesa Allen, Deborah Baker, Rhonda Brown Cotton, Katrina Yearby, First Lady Ann Sanders, Angela Hilson, Nikki Brown King, my hairstylist/sister friend Ericka Marshall, Yvonne Coulter, Robin Williams, Natasha Franklin, Carse Franklin III, Pastor Janard and First Lady Shunta Lakes, Mother Lakes and the Spirit of Victory daily prayer line family, Renee Jones and BTG family, Apostle Dr. Vanessa Burns and the Tuesday prayer line family, Kimica Lee, my former boss from Easter Seals Kathleen Hendericks, the University of Michigan Ann Arbor Hospital Staff, and so many others too numerous to name—people all across the entire country.

Six Months of Grace

I began chemo treatments from November 2022 through April 2023, every week on Thursday from 9:30 AM to 5 PM for 6 months straight. My son Colonel and daughter-in-law Amber drove 45 minutes to be by my side, supporting me throughout the cold capping process. They helped me change the cold caps every 20 minutes, even staying an hour after chemo to continue assisting in my effort to preserve my hair.

I was blessed to be surrounded by the love of my immediate family after each chemo session. I rested, and we always enjoyed good meals together, making those moments even more special.

The treatments were hard on my body, taking my 145-pound frame to 196 pounds. This was challenging to carry and look at daily. I would declare Deuteronomy 33:25: "Thy shoes shall be iron and brass; and as thy days, so shall thy strength be." I definitely needed to hold on to the word that "God is able and He won't fail," and recognize the great grace He provided me throughout every stage of my journey.

Overall, throughout the chemo, God carried me through, and the prayers on my behalf were life-changing. But the chemo drug called the Red Devil (Doxorubicin) and the immunotherapy drug Keytruda were too much for me, and I ended up in the hospital. My symptoms were shortness of breath, weakness, and I could barely get around. I also lost a halo of hair down to my scalp from the front to the back.

After leaving the hospital, I contacted the oncologist to tell him I no longer wanted to continue chemo, and he said if I stopped, I would die. I continued to counsel others and work throughout chemo and had reached a point where I said to God, "I am so tired of going through all this. I need some rest."

The Fight for My Very Life

On April 14th, I received a call from my nephrologist stating to go into the hospital for kidney dehydration, so I thought. I went into the hospital, and different things started happening to the point I started being delusional and incoherent. My son Colonel and daughter-in-love Amber had to activate my advance directive and take over making medical decisions for me because I couldn't. I had completely shut down and stopped eating.

Little did they know this was the beginning of a fight for my very life.

Later that month, I went into a coma from the middle of April 2023 until June 2023. During these 3 months, my son and daughter-in-law were by my side every day advocating with the healthcare team along with my mom and dad. The physicians treated me for some type of infection but couldn't determine what was wrong even after giving me every test possible.

During this time, my heart stopped twice, and God allowed them to restart my heart. (First miracle.)

The physician had a meeting with my son and daughter-in-love, recommending they place me into hospice because there was nothing they could do for me. My son believed this was not my end and that God was faithful to change this situation. He was determined to get me transferred to the University of Michigan Hospital. He faced obstacles to get this done, but God allowed a bed to become available.

Within 24 hours of being at U of M Hospital, God performed a miracle by allowing the physician to determine what was wrong with me and why I went into a coma.

I woke up out of that coma after 3 months—in 24 hours. Hallelujah, miracle-working God! (Second miracle.)

It was determined the chemo medication took all the cortisol out of my body and damaged my body's ability to produce cortisol. You can't live without cortisol, but God allowed me to go into a coma instead of dying. Glory, honor, and praise to God for His faithfulness toward me.

I'm thankful to my son and daughter-in-love for every sacrifice, driving daily from Auburn Hills, and most importantly, not giving up but continuing to believe and trust God. I'm grateful for everyone that prayed for me. God was so faithful—He got me to the hospital for something else to save me. I didn't pass away at home by myself or fall out dead somewhere. Even when things seemed at their worst, I realized there was always a greater purpose behind it all. (Third miracle.)

Rehab and Restoration

I had to go through rehab to walk again, cognitive restoration and strengthening, and relearning daily tasks. This was not an easy journey. One of the pastors from my church, Veotis Jones, reminded me of having an "evidence file." This was such encouragement because we all have evidence of something that seemed impossible and not likely for us to get through, but God allowed us to have a different outcome—which is the evidence file.

I've had an evidence file from the previous year of 2021 when I had a 3-brain bleed stroke and got up with no deficits within seven days and also walked without having rehab. Miracle-working and mighty God has given me great evidence of His power before, and the same God showed me mighty evidence through cancer, coma, and rehab. But God wasn't done showing me miracle signs and wonders.

I was transferred to Chelsea Hospital for rehab. God's word and (fourth miracle) got me through rehab in one week. Cognitively, I couldn't remember how to tell time from a clock and had to relearn how to tell time all over again. I also had to learn how to stop dragging my leg, walk with a walker, get up from bed and floor, bathe, clean myself, and coordinate my hands. God allowed me to complete it all in one week. This had not been done in rehab before.

I felt the enabling ability of the Holy Spirit daily through rehab. Once I left rehab, I also had in-home rehab for additional progression. I had to get a heart defibrillator monitor bag I carried daily.

More Battles, More Victories

On August 8, 2023, I had surgery to remove the cancer from both of my breasts—a double mastectomy—and lymph nodes. After the completion of surgery, an artery began bleeding, and the surgeon had to take me back to surgery to stop the bleeding.

Due to the numerous surgeries, anesthesia, and the decreased function of my kidneys, they eventually failed. As a result, I had to start dialysis three times a week. The recovery process from the double mastectomy and now weekly dialysis was a lot to process and deal with after getting through chemo and a coma with rehab.

I also had to begin radiation daily after my breasts were removed. Due to the cancer being metastasized in my lymph nodes, radiation was required. So just when I thought the fight was over, daily radiation, recovery from the double mastectomy, and three days of dialysis were only beginning.

This was not easy, but I'm grateful for the daily prayers of family, friends, and so many from church, prayer lines, and others from across the country. So many days, I continuously declared God's word over my life: "As my days, so shall my strength be," in the mighty name of Jesus.

I had to start radiation in December of 2023 through early February 2024 daily, along with follow-up appointments and dialysis three days a week. I had several surgeries for dialysis and even heart defibrillator surgery.

The Report I Prayed For

The best appointment was the day of my PET scan when my results came back with no evidence of recurrent or residual cancer—just as God promised. He was faithful, and He didn't fail. I am healed! Now that's some undeniable evidence screaming on my behalf.

I'm so grateful I was able to host a Praise Celebration in April 2024 to glorify God for the great and mighty things He has done. His many signs, miracles, and wonders worked on my behalf repeatedly.

The Prescription That Changes Everything

If you're facing cancer or any illness, my cousin Angela Vaughn shared the best prescription that was powerful and life-changing for me. With so many people praying for me, I firmly believe in the power of calling on the saints to pray.

"Is anyone among you sick? Let him call for the elders of the church, and let them pray over him, anointing him with oil in the name of the Lord. And the prayer of faith will save the sick, and the Lord will RAISE HIM UP. And if he has committed sins, he will be forgiven." James 5:14-16 (KJV)

The word in Matthew 18:20 also reminds us that where two or three are gathered in His name, the Lord promises to be in the midst of them. So, if one can chase a thousand, then two can chase—COME ON SAY IT WITH ME—ten thousand!

God has given us authority to speak to EVERY situation, and in my case, it was back-to-back healing we were calling for! I am a walking and moving testimony of God's work in the earth when we use our authority.

Whenever the doctors reported about what was going on with me, Ketesa, Lesia, Deborah, and so many others were attacking it in prayer on one accord. That's why it's important to be specific about what's going on, so the saints can be saying (bombarding heaven) the same thing.

I was literally raised from my deathbed. Some of y'all didn't see what my family saw! Even when the healing began, the devil still tried to take my mind, but guess what—that didn't work either.

Praise God for my life! LOOK AT GOD!

> *"And God raised us up with Christ and seated us with him in the heavenly realms in Christ Jesus."*
> **Ephesians 2:6 (ESV)**

Sister, you are not just a survivor—you are more than a conqueror. You are a walking miracle. You are living proof that God is faithful and He will not fail.

Walk in your miracle. Declare your victory. And when the enemy tries to remind you of your past, you remind him of his future!

God is able, and He won't fail

Dear Sister,

Please know that you are valued and that you are loved. When God created you, He really did a phenomenal job. Cancer is a pothole in God's street of life. You will fill that pothole up with God's grace, love, mercy, strength, power, humility, fortitude, and courage to continue to have a sound mind, that God has given you this task, so that you can come out of it to let those sisters that are coming behind you know that His light shines in you, and through you forever.

                Renee

My Journey through Endometrial/Uterine Cancer

Authored By: Renee Conley

June 15, 2023, started like any other day in my recovery from left knee replacement surgery. I was focused on healing, following doctor's orders, and getting back to my normal routine. I had no idea that my body was harboring a secret that would change everything.

Two days after my knee surgery, strange things began happening that I couldn't explain. I was drinking large quantities of water—more than usual—but when it came time for the nurse to measure my urine output, there wasn't enough to record. This happened several times, and I could see the confusion on the medical staff's faces.

Finally, the nurse asked me, "Ms. Conley, are you emptying your urinal?"

I looked at her like she had lost her mind. "I don't work here! Why would I do that?"

She laughed and said, "Then where is it all going?"

I had no idea. But her question sent a chill through me because I realized something was very wrong with my body.

They brought an ultrasound machine into the room to investigate, and I heard the nurse say words that I'll never forget: "You have 999 kilograms of liquid on you."

999 kilograms. Let that sink in for a moment.

I was immediately sent for an emergency ultrasound scan. The technician performing the scan had a look on her face that I couldn't read, but it wasn't reassuring. "I don't know what that is," she said. "Your doctor will call you with the results."

And just like that, this rollercoaster ride began.

The Discovery That Changed Everything

The doctor referred me to my OB-GYN, who attempted to perform a biopsy. However, what should have been a routine procedure turned into something much more serious. I ended up needing emergency surgery because, unbeknownst to any of us, a tumor was blocking the entrance to my vagina.

When they told me the size of this tumor, I couldn't process it at first. The tumor was the size of a four-month-old baby. A baby. Growing inside me without my knowledge.

Looking back, there had been signs I didn't recognize. When you touched my stomach, the sides were very soft, but the middle was hard. You could even move it up and down and feel that you were shifting my uterus. I had attributed these changes to weight gain, to getting older, to anything but cancer.

That 999 kilograms of liquid I had accumulated? It turned out to be the equivalent of four 2-liter bottles of blood. My body had been trying to tell me something was wrong, but I didn't speak its language.

There was another tumor they discovered—one they couldn't reach because it was too large. They would have to shrink it before they could remove it through surgery. This was the beginning of my new life, though I didn't know it yet.

I was diagnosed with endometrial cancer.

It all happened so quickly that I didn't even have time to process everything. One moment I was recovering from knee surgery, and the next I was facing a cancer diagnosis with tumors the size of babies growing inside me.

The Questions That Haunted Me

I was scared and had no idea what any of this meant for my future. My mind immediately went to the darkest places. Should I start preparing for my funeral? Who would help my children with my last wishes? What is endometrial cancer, and how did I get it?

These were the questions I bombarded the doctors with, but I realized I needed to find my own answers too. I couldn't just sit passively and let this happen to me. I needed to understand what I was fighting.

I learned that endometrial cancer is cancer of the lining of the uterus, also known as the womb. It's also referred to as uterine cancer. But knowing the clinical definition didn't help me understand why this was happening to me.

So I began researching. I talked to healthcare professionals. I reached out to the Cancer Society. I needed to understand not just what endometrial cancer was, but how it had taken root in my body without me knowing.

The Weight of Truth

What I discovered about the risk factors hit me like a physical blow. The number one risk factor for endometrial cancer is obesity. Other risk factors included increased age (75% of women diagnosed with endometrial cancer are postmenopausal), the use of estrogen hormones without progesterone, hypertension, diabetes, the use of tamoxifen, and a family history of colon, uterine, or ovarian cancer.

I felt deeply upset with myself because my weight had been a lifelong struggle. Eight years ago, I weighed 400 pounds. It's hard for some people to believe when I share my weight challenges, but that was my reality. Through my research, I learned that my risk factor of obesity was compounded by decreased physical activity. Carrying extra weight led to higher circulating levels of estrogen, which significantly increased my risk for endometrial cancer.

I was mortified. What had I done to myself?

But then I had to stop and redirect that self-blame. Yes, my weight had been a contributing factor, but cancer isn't a punishment for poor choices. Cancer doesn't discriminate based on whether you "deserve" it or not. And beating myself up wasn't going to help me fight this disease.

> "She is clothed with strength and dignity;
> she can laugh at the days to come."
> **Proverbs 31:25 (ESV)**

I had to find strength in the truth, not shame in the circumstances.

The Signs I Missed

It's important to understand that each person diagnosed with endometrial cancer experiences different symptoms. Some may not have the same warning signs as others. For instance, I did not experience any bleeding or spotting, which are the most commonly discussed symptoms.

However, I did notice a discharge that had a brownish color. Sometimes this discharge can appear pinkish or brownish, and for women who are postmenopausal like me, any discharge should be investigated.

I had not had a period in over nine years. Because I am older and had already gone through menopause, this discharge turned out to be a crucial symptom of endometrial cancer. For younger women, irregular periods or heavier bleeding during cycles can be warning signs. It's crucial to report any abnormal changes in your menstrual cycle to your doctor.

I had no idea about any of this. I thought that because I got regular check-ups, yearly mammograms, and Pap smears, I was covered. I was diligent about my health screenings, or so I thought. Unfortunately, routine Pap smears don't screen for endometrial cancer—they primarily detect cervical cancer.

This was a wake-up call about how much I didn't know about my own body and the cancers that could affect it.

A Painful Truth About Survival

As I researched my diagnosis, I stumbled upon statistics that broke my heart and ignited a fire in me. I wondered whether more African American women were experiencing endometrial cancer compared to Caucasian women, and what I found was devastating.

According to the American Cancer Society, the United States is projected to see 67,880 new cases of endometrial cancer in 2024, with approximately

13,250 women expected to die from cancers of the uterus. This cancer is more common in Black women than in White women. Over the past decade, the incidence rate has increased by about 1% per year in White women and by 2%-3% in other ethnic and racial groups.

But here's the statistic that haunts me: Black women are more likely to die from endometrial or uterine cancer.

Why? The number one difference is treatment access. Black and Hispanic women are less likely to receive surgery as a treatment for cancer. Barriers to treatment often stem from systemic inequities, including lower socioeconomic status, which is usually shaped by neighborhoods, health insurance access, education, and income levels.

It is 2024, yet this inequity still persists. This is heartbreaking to witness in America. No one wants to believe this is still happening, but it is. And it's not just statistics—it's real women, real families, real lives being affected by a system that doesn't value all lives equally.

As I went through my own experience, I often wondered how I could help someone else who might not have the support system I was fortunate to have. How many women were getting diagnosed later because they didn't have access to quality healthcare? How many were facing this battle alone?

My Treatment Journey

After the initial shock of diagnosis, my treatment plan became my new reality. The tumors were too large for immediate surgical removal, so I had to undergo chemotherapy first to shrink them. This was not the quick fix I had hoped for—this was going to be a long battle.

The chemotherapy was harder than I expected. Not just physically, but emotionally. Each treatment cycle reminded me that my body had betrayed me, that despite my efforts to take care of myself through regular check-ups, cancer had still found a way in.

But I also learned something important during those long hours in the chemo chair: I was stronger than I knew. Each treatment was a small victory, each day I woke up was a gift. I started seeing the treatments not as something being done to me, but as something I was actively doing to fight for my life.

The surgical removal came later, after the tumors had shrunk enough to be safely extracted. The day of surgery, I remember feeling both terrified and hopeful. Terrified because any surgery carries risks, but hopeful because this was my chance to get the cancer out of my body once and for all.

Recovery was slow but steady. My body had been through so much—the cancer, the chemotherapy, the surgery—and it needed time to heal. I had to learn patience with myself and trust the process.

Living as a Survivor

Today, as I write this, I am cancer-free. But survivorship brings its own challenges that no one really prepares you for. Every follow-up appointment brings anxiety. Every unusual feeling in my body makes me wonder if the cancer has returned. The fear of recurrence is real and constant.

But I've also found purpose in my pain. My research into endometrial cancer and health disparities has become more than academic interest—it's become my mission. I want every woman, especially every Black woman, to know the signs and symptoms I missed. I want them to advocate for themselves in ways I didn't know I needed to.

I've learned that being a cancer survivor means more than just being disease-free. It means living with the knowledge of your mortality while choosing to embrace life fully. It means using your experience to help others navigate their own journeys.

"And we know that in all things God works for the good of those who love him, who have been called according to his purpose." Romans 8:28 (ESV)

What Every Woman Needs to Know

The National Cancer Institute reports that there is no known way to prevent endometrial cancer completely. However, we can lower our risk factors through awareness and action.

Here's what I wish I had known before my diagnosis:

Know the Risk Factors: Obesity, age, hormone therapy, diabetes, hypertension, and family history all play a role. If you have multiple risk factors like I did, be extra vigilant about symptoms.

Understand the Symptoms: Any unusual bleeding or discharge, especially after menopause, should be investigated immediately. Don't assume it's "just aging" or "just stress."

Advocate for Yourself: If something feels wrong, push for answers. Don't let anyone dismiss your concerns. Trust your body—it often knows something is wrong before tests can detect it.

Address Health Disparities: If you're a Black woman, be especially proactive about your healthcare. Ask questions, seek second opinions, and don't accept substandard care.

Know Your Family History: Understanding your family's cancer history can help you and your doctor make informed decisions about screening and prevention.

A Message to My Sisters

To every woman reading this, especially my Black sisters: your life matters. Your health matters. Your voice matters.

Don't let anyone minimize your symptoms or dismiss your concerns. Don't let socioeconomic barriers prevent you from seeking the care you deserve. Don't let fear keep you from getting the screenings that could save your life.

If you're currently fighting endometrial cancer, know that you are not alone. The journey is difficult, but you are stronger than you know. Take it one day at a time, one treatment at a time, one victory at a time.

And if you're a survivor like me, consider how you can use your experience to help others. Share your story. Educate your community. Advocate for better healthcare access. Be the voice for women who don't yet have one.

My diagnosis taught me that my body had been trying to communicate with me for months, but I didn't know how to listen. Now I'm committed to helping other women learn that language—the language of their own bodies, the language of self-advocacy, the language of survival.

"She watches over the affairs of her household and does not eat the bread of idleness. Her children arise and call her blessed; her husband also, and he praises her." Proverbs 31:27-28 (ESV)

BLACK WOMEN SURVIVING SURVIVORSHIP

We are watchers, protectors, advocates—for ourselves and for each other. This is how we change the statistics. This is how we save lives.

This is how we turn our pain into purpose.

Your life is worth fighting for. Your story matters. And your survival can be someone else's hope.

Dear Sister,

I need you to know right now—you are not alone in this. I may not know every detail of your story, but I know the weight of this fight, and I honor the strength it takes just to keep showing up each day. None of us asked for this journey, but here you are, still standing, still fighting, still breathing. That alone is courage. Hold on to your faith and remember that God has not forgotten you. Even when it feels dark, His hand is on you, carrying you through and covering you with His peace, healing, and strength. My prayer is that as you read my story, you find comfort, hope, and a reminder that we are not just survivors—we are warriors, chosen and equipped by God to keep moving forward.

Sabrina

Embracing Self-Care: A Guide to Thriving After Breast Cancer Treatment

Authored By: Sabrina Thomas

I was not prepared for what 2023 had to offer me.

On February 5, 2023, I noticed a lump in my breast when trying on clothes for an upcoming cruise. Just like that, my world shifted without me even knowing it yet. On February 24, 2023, I was diagnosed with Stage 2B breast cancer, Invasive Ductal carcinoma, meaning the cancer was growing at a fast pace and I needed to seek treatment immediately.

As I waited for results from ultrasounds, biopsy, and blood work, I convinced myself that I did not have cancer. First, I thought, it doesn't run in my family and secondly, I thought, okay, I already have a special needs adult son I am caring for. God doesn't put more on you than you can bear, so I am good. I can't have anything else on my plate. He loves me and he wouldn't do that to me.

But on February 24th, when I went to get my results and walked into that conference room, I already knew I had cancer. It was the energy in the room, the tone, and the expression on their faces.

Dammmmmmmmmmmm.

It was a surreal moment filled with sadness and hurt. I felt a sudden deliberate attack by my own body. I felt like everything just stopped. I really don't remember hearing anything else after I was told I had cancer. I just cried.

The diagnosis didn't really hit me until later that evening and early the next morning. I had a weekend out of town planned and I didn't want to go, but I did. It was an emotional weekend, but I think I needed it. When you get a cancer diagnosis, life doesn't stop. It just changes. I still had to live.

I remember the next morning calling my cousin and she was at church. She ran and told the pastor, and he got on the phone and prayed for me. It really touched me, the words he said. That prayer gave me peace in that moment.

> *"Having cancer does make you try to be better at everything you do and enjoy every moment. It changes you forever. But it can be a positive change."*
> **- Jaclyn Smith**

The Wrestling and the Questions

After the initial shock, the questions came flooding in. I've overcome so much in my life; I don't want to fight this battle too. What about my sons? What about Omar? Who's going to take care of him? God, why? Did I do something wrong? Am I doing something wrong? Is this my karma?

Cancer has taught me that it's an emotional rollercoaster—hands-in-the-air on the emotionally good days and hands-over-my-eyes on the emotionally bad days. A cancer diagnosis changes your whole perspective on life. You grow to appreciate the little things. You learn that patience and faith are how you survive.

After going through all the emotions, the tears, and the questions, I've come to a place of peace. You know that peace that transcends all understanding.

If you know me, then you know I'm not afraid to fight. Not because I'm so great, but because that is just who I am. I will fight with all the tools available to me—surgery, chemotherapy, diet, but most of all prayer and the Word of God.

The Hardest Conversation

The one thing I dreaded most was telling my oldest son. I didn't have to worry about telling my youngest son because he wouldn't understand due to his intellectual disability. I put it off, but I had to tell him, and I chose to do it at my mom's house.

There are no perfect or right or wrong words when you're telling your child you have cancer. I finally told him, and his facial expression was one I will never forget. In that moment and for moments after, I just wanted him to be supported, because I knew I was going through and trying to process this myself. I couldn't be that person for him right then. My mom was able to check on him daily. My close friends and their children became his support system when he needed it.

We talk almost daily now. We were already close anyway; the situation just made us closer in a different way.

"Cast all your anxiety on him because he cares for you."
- 1 Peter 5:7

When One Battle Became Two

Everything was moving so fast—appointments, blood work, biopsies, ultrasounds. I was having so much anxiety because I was so overwhelmed. I was getting prepared for a lumpectomy, so I needed an MRI. When I had the MRI done, they saw something suspicious on my left breast. I was like, "Really, God?"

Well, the results came in and I had cancer in both breasts. I just broke inside. It was like the world just stopped. I was numb. I instantly felt like my body—my breasts—were trying to kill me, and honestly, I just wanted them gone. I didn't want them anymore. I wanted to live; I just wanted to live, and if I had cancer in both breasts, that wasn't good. It's like you have double chances of dying, the odds stacked against me twice. I just wanted surgery right away. I just wanted the cancer out of my body.

I had some major decisions to make and time was not on my side, but I honestly already knew in my mind what I wanted to do. Wowwwww, this is really my life...

I had breast cancer in both my breasts. Jesus be a fence!

Whatever is weighing on your heart, give it to God and feel the weight lift off your shoulders.

Finding My Way: Prayer and Processing

At the beginning, all I could say to people was "I am praying and processing" because I was trying to process this whole thing and pray about it as well. My faith has been tested several times through this journey. I started speaking about healing over my life and I started to pray differently.

Prayer became my lifeline. It's the best way to bring forth a solution and peace with any situation. Most of us realize that our own strength is not always enough to get through some of the situations that this life brings. At those difficult times, we must call on God for extra strength and for His strength to help sustain us when our own strength fails. Sometimes our own strength is just not enough. Most times for me, it isn't.

The real test in your faith is when you feel like your prayers aren't being heard or answered. However, if you are patient and faithful enough to keep going even when you can't see what's coming, you will look up one day and realize that the wait was worth it and necessary to prepare you for what you prayed for. In the meantime, keep believing and working like your next breakthrough could be just around the corner.

"He says, 'Be still, and know that I am God.'"
- Psalm 46:10

The Mental Battle: Mindset is Everything

Getting a cancer diagnosis doesn't just affect the person who got the diagnosis but the entire family and close friends as well. After a few days of feeling sorry for myself and questioning God, I prayed for healing, clarity, and peace! Breast cancer forced me to step back and put things in perspective. It forced me to start taking better care of my physical and mental health.

Cancer is very much mental. The mindset plays a crucial role in the recovery and overall well-being of breast cancer survivors. I learned that having a positive mindset and attitude after breast cancer treatment involves a combination of self-compassion, proactive health management, and a focus on living a fulfilling life.

While a positive mindset is beneficial, it's also important to acknowledge that it's normal to experience a range of emotions, including fear, anger, and sadness. Acceptance of these emotions is part of the healing process. It's not an easy process, but it's a process nonetheless. Keep moving through it.

According to the American Cancer Society, survivors with a positive mindset report better physical, emotional, and social functioning. A positive mindset helps in building resilience, allowing survivors to cope better with the emotional and psychological challenges post-treatment.

> *"Cancer can take away all of my physical abilities. It cannot touch my mind, it cannot touch my heart, and it cannot touch my soul."*
> **- Jim Valvano**

Learning to Thrive: My Self-Care Revolution

This journey has been arduous, marked by pain, fear, and uncertainty, but it has also been a testament to my resilience, faith, and determination. God literally restored and revived my life this past year, and he gifted me a most powerful testimony.

Through this experience, I discovered that moving forward emotionally after breast cancer treatment is challenging, but with time and intentional self-care, it is possible to find a new sense of normalcy and well-being. Everyone's journey is unique, and it's important to find what works best for you and to prioritize your emotional well-being as you move forward.

Here's what I learned about thriving after treatment:

Physical Health Became My Foundation Regular follow-up appointments with my oncologist became vital for monitoring my recovery and catching any potential issues early. I learned that a balanced diet rich in fruits, vegetables, lean proteins, and whole grains could support my body's healing process. Gentle, regular exercise helped improve my physical strength and energy levels, though I always consulted my doctor before starting any new exercise regimen.

Rest and sleep became sacred to me—I had to ensure I got enough to help my body heal and reduce fatigue. If you're at risk for lymphedema, following your healthcare provider's advice on prevention and management is crucial. Taking prescribed medications as directed and discussing any side effects with your healthcare provider becomes part of your new normal.

Emotional and Mental Health Required Intentional Work Speaking with a counselor helped me process my emotions and cope with the stress of recovery. Joining support groups provided a sense of community and understanding from others who had gone through similar experiences. Practices such as mindfulness, meditation, and deep-breathing exercises helped reduce stress and improve mental clarity.

I learned to focus on the present and appreciate each day, which helped reduce anxiety about the future. Keeping a gratitude journal shifted my focus to positive aspects of my life. Positive affirmations became powerful tools—statements like "I am strong," "I am resilient," and "I am healing" reinforced my faith and self-image.

Social Support Became My Lifeline I learned to keep open lines of communication with family and friends, letting them know how they could support me. I had to avoid stressful situations and focus on activities that brought me joy and relaxation. Staying connected with friends and family became crucial for emotional well-being.

Setting boundaries became essential—I learned to say no to situations or people that drained my energy or negatively impacted my self-esteem. Surrounding myself with positivity meant spending time with people who uplifted and supported me.

Becoming a Warrior Queen

My journey through breast cancer was a battle fought with courage, strength, and an unyielding spirit. Now that I am on the other side of treatment, I walk with a new purpose and a renewed sense of self.

I am a warrior, a Black queen who faced the storm head-on and emerged stronger, more resilient. My mindset is my greatest armor, a shield forged in the fires of adversity. Each day, I choose to see the beauty in life, to celebrate my victories, no matter how small.

Every day I embrace my new body, cherishing its resilience and strength. I know that healing is not just physical; it is a journey of the soul. Self-love and self-care have become my mantras. I speak words of affirmation that uplift my spirit: "I am strong. I am beautiful. I am enough. I am cancer-free." These words have become my anthem, a reminder of my worth and strength.

You are a warrior too, and it's time to own it. Wear that invisible crown and remind yourself daily of your strength. Whether it's bold red lipstick or a stunning outfit, dress up and step out like the queen you are. Your body has been through a marathon, not a sprint. Give yourself permission to rest and recharge.

Every single day is a victory. Celebrate your milestones, no matter how small—each one is worth a toast. Celebrate your journey, your strength, and your incredible resilience.

> *"We have two options, medically and emotionally: give up or fight like hell."*
> **- Lance Armstrong**

Practical Wisdom for Your Journey

Reclaim Your Confidence Cancer tried to shake your confidence, but it failed. You are stronger than ever. Embrace your scars—they're badges of honor. Flaunt your fabulousness. Whether it's rocking a new hairstyle or sporting that bold lipstick, own your new look. Confidence is your best accessory.

Listen to Your Body Post-treatment fatigue is real—I'm experiencing this right now. Listen to your body and give it the rest it needs. But when you're ready, find energizing activities that make you feel alive. Dance around your living room, take a brisk walk, or try yoga. Rest is crucial, but so is living vibrantly.

Nourish Your Temple Your body is a temple, and it's time to treat it like one. Fill your plate with nutritious, colorful foods that fuel your spirit. Think vibrant salads, fresh fruits, and lean proteins. And let's be real—don't deny yourself the occasional treat. Balance is key, and you deserve it.

Create Your New Normal Life after treatment can feel like uncharted territory. Embrace it! Create new routines that bring you joy and structure. Rediscover hobbies or dive into new ones. Your new normal is all about living your best life.

Honor Your Emotions Emotional ups and downs are part of the journey. Acknowledge your feelings—they're valid. Seek support from friends and family. Practice mindfulness and self-compassion. You've been through a lot, and it's okay to feel all the feelings. Own your emotions with pride.

Chase Your Dreams Now's the time to chase those dreams. What have you always wanted to do? Travel, start a new hobby, change careers? Go for it! The world is your oyster, and there's no time like the present to pursue your passions.

"You gain strength, courage, and confidence by every experience in which you really stop to look fear in the face."
- Eleanor Roosevelt

Living as a Beacon of Hope

There will be challenges, but my spirit is unbreakable, and my heart is full of hope. Having a positive mindset is not just a choice for me—it's my only option.

Life after breast cancer treatment is a landscape of change. My body bears the scars of surgery, the effects of chemotherapy, and the fatigue from treatment. Yet each scar is a badge of courage, a symbol of the battles I have won. I embrace my new normal, understanding that healing is a continuous process, both physically and emotionally.

Resilience is not just about bouncing back; it's about growing through adversity. It takes time to nurture mental and emotional health. Therapy, support groups, and connecting with fellow survivors have become my safe spaces, providing room to share fears and triumphs. I practice self-compassion and allow myself to feel and process the complex emotions that accompany this journey.

Breast cancer has changed me, but it has also illuminated my passions and purpose. Empowered by my experience, I feel called to give back. Advocacy has become part of my life, whether through sharing my story, participating in breast cancer awareness initiatives, or supporting others who are just beginning their journey. My voice is a powerful tool for change, helping to raise awareness and provide hope.

One day you will appreciate everything you had to endure to become the person you are today. It sounds simple, but it's not. It is only when we have overcome life's challenges that we realize how strong we really are. Spiritual muscles are usually built when we are in crisis, and those same spiritual muscles allow us to do the "impossible."

You Can't Give Up Now

The path ahead is one of hope and possibility. I know that challenges may still arise, but I will face them with the resilience that has carried me this far. This journey through breast cancer has forged a spirit of strength, courage, and unwavering determination.

Moving forward after breast cancer treatment is a personal and unique journey. Be patient with yourself, seek support when needed, and prioritize your well-being as you navigate this new chapter in your life. Practicing self-love is an ongoing process, and it's important to be patient and gentle with yourself as you navigate this journey.

What God has for you, no one can take from you—I learned that years ago. It doesn't mean you won't have tough times while you are waiting for your prayers to be answered, but it does mean God will carry you through it all. Your part is to know and believe you can do all things through God, who strengthens you.

If you don't have a prayer life now, I urge you to get one. Prayer should be in your daily routine. When I start my day with prayer, I feel a sense of peace.

It may be a rough season for you right now; however, try to see what you can learn from it. There is always a lesson to be learned.

I am a survivor, a beacon of resilience. My story is a testament to the power of the human spirit to overcome, to heal, and to thrive. And as I move forward, I carry the knowledge that I can face anything that comes my way with grace, dignity, and an unbreakable will.

My life is a beacon of hope, and I will continue to inspire others as I share my story of resilience through my breast cancer journey.

Thank you, Lord, for being there for me and allowing me to cry out to you in my times of need. I know that the situation is in Your hands, and I trust You.

This has been a journey, but with God and His grace and favor, I am still alive and thriving. God has proven over and over again that there is power in prayer. If there were any questions before now regarding the divine path orchestrated for me, there are no more. I am even more committed to doing those things which God has ordained for my life, and He will continuously receive the honor, glory, and praise that He deserves.

Dear sister,

I wrote this because I want you to know to keep the faith and stay strong. You are a beautiful woman of God—stay motivated, never be ashamed of your scars. Stay strong because you're a survivor.

In case nobody told you this yet, you are an overcomer! You push through. You're still here. Still standing. Just stay in faith.

God bless you.

                                              Sandra

Thriving and Surviving

Authored by Sandra Ewing

Imagine waking up and your breasts are hurting, and you're like, *what's going on?* This was just before Christmas in 2012, when I first noticed something wasn't right. I called my sister and said my breasts were hurting really badly. She said to put some heat on them, so I did the next day, but they were still hurting.

I told my sister I needed to get an exam. I made the call and let them know that my breasts were hurting and I needed to make an appointment, only to hear, "We are not making any appointments." I'm like, what? I need a mammogram. I'm in pain.

At that time in my life, I had the Ingham County health plan, and they were not covering mammograms. So, I'm like, wow, really, what's going on? I'm my own advocate, so I called the number on the back of my card, and my doctor was able to get me an appointment. I thank God for being my own advocate.

When management found out I couldn't get an appointment with Ingham County, they said I would receive phone call after phone call. I was told this would never happen again, and they were very sorry. But I had already learned my first lesson: you have to fight for your healthcare.

The Shocking Discovery

Well, I got my mammogram, and they said I needed to get an ultrasound as well. I'm getting the ultrasound, and they said they needed to do a biopsy. "We see something," they told me. My heart dropped, and I said, "Okay."

I felt the lump, but wasn't sure what it meant. I was surprised how quickly the doctors got me right in for all my tests. My doctor said I had a lump, but not to worry—it was probably nothing. I kept my faith high, believing it to be "nothing."

So, I had to go see a surgical oncologist, and we talked about the breast cancer diagnosis and what had to be done. I also had to go to a planning class about my surgery, where I got to meet the other doctors, and they all had to examine me.

Then a lady doctor comes in and says, "Can I check you?" I said yes. She said, "Lift your arm up," and wow, she said, "I feel a lump on your left side." I'm like, really? So, I said, "What's next?" She said I had to go get another biopsy.

On January 21, I had a biopsy. It was very painful because they had to go deep with the needle, only to find out it was cancer. So not only did I have a lump in my breast, but I also had a lump under my arm. The plan of action became, "What's next? OMG, emotions everywhere."

I had one more appointment to talk about what they were going to do, and my surgery was scheduled for January 30, 2013. It was time to get the cancer removed from my body.

Surgery and Treatment

One thing I can say is that I had a beautiful support system. All my friends and family were there for me. I know God is good, and I knew everything was going to be okay. I kept my faith.

I had a lumpectomy on my left side and a lymph node dissection. I had 12 lymph nodes removed because the cancer had spread to my lymph nodes. I was officially diagnosed with an "Invasive Ductal Carcinoma, Estrogen Receptor-positive Tumor." They staged me at 3A, and HER-2 positive.

I thank God that I made it through the surgery, and I was very nervous about my next step. I was told I would have to do chemotherapy and radiation. Emotions were running all over because you hear so many stories about chemotherapy, but I kept my faith in God, and I knew everything was going to be okay.

I had to make an appointment to get a port put in to start my chemotherapy. Emotions everywhere, not knowing what to expect, but I continued to keep my faith.

After healing from surgery and taking chemotherapy classes, it was time to start chemotherapy. My nerves were all over the place. I didn't know what would happen next, but I continued to keep my faith and pray that everything would be okay.

I started chemotherapy on March 27, 2013, and continued until August 28, 2013. I continued taking Herceptin because of being HER-2 positive for a year, every three weeks. On May 21, 2014, I completed that treatment.

But let me tell you that chemotherapy was no joke. I did two different kinds of chemotherapy, and one of them was called "the red devil." When I say the red devil made you sick—I was at the point in my life where I could not look at anything red. It made me very, very ill.

My emotions were running wild because going through chemotherapy takes a toll on your body. A lot of things happen to your body, including losing your hair. I know it's nothing but hair, but at that time, I didn't look at it like that. I was devastated when my hair fell out. I cried. But I had to realize it's just hair and it will grow back. I had more important things to worry about than hair because I was sick.

Chemotherapy made me so sick. All I could do was sleep. I had to take pills every 6 to 8 hours, but I was still ill and could not function. The only thing you can do is pray to God that you get through it. Stay strong and never give up. Keep fighting the fight.

Radiation and Recovery

After I finished my chemotherapy, I had to start radiation treatments from October 9, 2013, to November 2013. Radiation was very different. You had to go every day. It was easy, but it did make you tired, and I got burned really badly.

At my appointment, I was told I would have to take a five-year cancer pill, so I was put on Letrozole 2.5 mg daily from November 2013 to November 2017.

My emotions were still running everywhere, despite the fact that I had breast cancer and was going through chemotherapy and radiation, not feeling well, and not knowing how to live my life. My doctor said I didn't need to worry about all that and to live life to the fullest. I said, "You're exactly right!" So, I went on living my life the best way I knew how.

Well, after having radiation, I experienced swelling in my arm and hand, only to find out I had lymphedema. Of course, my mindset was, "What's next?" So, I had to go to physical therapy to get wraps for my arm and wear a compression garment on my arm and hand.

I went to physical therapy three times a week, getting massages and wraps until everything was under control, but I was told I would have to wear a garment on my arm and hand for the rest of my life because of the swelling from lymphedema.

> *"I can do all things through Christ who strengthens me."*
> **- Philippians 4:13 (ESV)**

The Return: Battle Number Two

I went on living my life to the fullest, not worrying about anything, not talking about it, just living life like I never had breast cancer. Then in July 2017, my breasts were hurting again, and I'm like, "There's no way. There's no way."

I had a mammogram on July 28, 2017, and it showed an irregular mass, so I had to have an ultrasound-guided biopsy again. Yes, the cancer had returned. I was devastated. My emotions ran all over the place because I didn't know how to tell my children that my cancer had returned. It was invasive intraductal carcinoma, ER positive, HER2 negative.

When that happened, I had to go in for a CT scan and a bone scan to make sure I didn't have metastatic disease, and everything came back negative. Thank God!

But I had made my decision. I told the doctors, "She's sick," referring to my breast. "She needs to come off." That's when I said I needed a mastectomy. I told my husband, "If you want to leave me, you can, but she's coming off because she's sick." He said, "I love you and don't worry about that. Everything is going to be fine."

I had a left mastectomy on September 13, 2017. When I tell you after surgery, I was in pain—I was in so much pain. I had drains hanging. It was horrible, but I made it through.

My granddaughter said, "Nanny, we're gonna get through this, so don't stress and don't worry. Everything is going to be okay." When she told me that, I looked at her and said, "You know what? You're exactly right. We are going to get through this, and everything is going to be okay." When a nine-year-old tells you that and she understands, the only thing you can do is be okay because God was in control.

After going back to the doctors, after my mastectomy, and hearing from them, I was told I would have to do chemotherapy again. So, I had to do four rounds of chemotherapy, and I completed that on November 19, 2017. I was told they would change my five-year breast cancer pill to Tamoxifen 20 mg as of July 11, 2018.

After completing my chemotherapy and learning to live life with one breast, I opted out of having reconstructive surgery. I told myself I had been through enough surgeries, and I didn't want to go through that.

The Unexpected Challenge

The hardest part of going through breast cancer and having to live with lymphedema was having a job, because when your job is not educated enough about those things, you can be mistreated without understanding how lymphedema affects your body and what you can and cannot do.

I will say I was my own advocate. I did what I needed to do to keep working until I hurt my shoulder, and that caused more problems because it was on the left side, where I had breast cancer. I opted for years not to have my shoulder done because I had a tear in my rotator cuff and needed surgery. I had to talk to my oncologist, and he said it should be okay, but we really didn't know for sure.

In March 2022, I went in and had my shoulder looked at, and it could not be fixed because I needed a whole shoulder replacement. Because of the lymphedema and the breast cancer, there was no way I could get that done, so I was not able to return to work. That brought more stress and heartache.

The Third Battle: When Miracle Meets Medicine

Only to find out months later, I was in pain again on my left side. I'm thinking, "There's no way I could have breast cancer again because my breast is gone." So, I called the doctor on August 23, 2022.

I went in for a CT scan on August 26, 2022, and the area of concern was in my left latissimus dorsi with intramuscular invasion measuring 5.8 cm x 3.2 cm with peripheral nodules.

So, I'm like, "What does that mean? I don't understand." My nerves were bad—like, what's going on? They said I had to have a biopsy, and it had to be done by CT scan to find the correct spot because it was so deep. My nerves were all over the place because I didn't know what to think. I'm crying, I'm crying, I'm crying, like, "This can't be happening again." I was thinking I had done something to my shoulder, and this caused the cancer to come back. I was just a nervous wreck.

On September 12, 2022, I was scheduled for my biopsy of the left latissimus dorsi. When my pathology came back, it showed I had metastatic carcinoma, ER positive, HER2 negative, and this was staged as oligometastatic disease.

Once again, my nerves were bad when I went to the doctor and got these results. He said it was breast cancer all over again, and I'm like, "How?" He said it just came back in a different part of my body, but it's breast cancer. I was just devastated.

I was like, "What's the plan of action?" I never lost my faith in God because I knew everything would be okay. One thing my grandmother said—she prayed to God and He told her everything was going to be fine. I was in agreement with my grandmother because we walk by faith and not by sight.

The Treatment Plan

I went to see my oncologist, and he said he had a plan of action. I would have to start doing chemotherapy every Monday for 12 weeks, and I would do two different kinds of chemotherapy and Herceptin as well. I was like, "Okay, I'm ready to get this started." Keeping my faith.

After doing 12 weeks of chemo, I completed it on December 22, 2022. My oncologist said I had to go in for a CT scan of my chest and pelvis with contrast to make sure nothing had spread anywhere else.

After doing the 12 weeks of chemo every Monday, the nodular mass had shrunk down to 9mm, which was great, and there was no evidence of metastasis. I'm giving God all the praise. Thank you, Jesus. It had shrunk because I was told it was the size of a tangerine, and surgery would have been difficult, so that's why they went with chemotherapy first.

The Miracle

My oncologist told me that I needed to meet with the breast cancer surgeon because he felt like the mass needed to be removed, so I would have to be scheduled for surgery. The breast cancer doctor sent me to a radiologist to put a marker in so he would know exactly where he needed to go when he was getting ready for surgery.

I went in to see the radiologist as they were prepping me. She said, "I don't see nothing." I'm like, "What?" She said, "Let me go get the radiologist so he can double-check." When I tell you—nothing, it was gone. God is so good. They could not believe it was gone, but I knew it was nothing but God. I kept my faith. I kept pressing. That chemotherapy dissolved that tumor all the way out of my body.

The doctor said that never happens. You have to have surgery or radiation to the area where the tumor is, but when I tell you, God is so good—no surgery, no radiation.

> *"And Jesus said unto him, If thou canst believe, all things are possible to him that believeth."*
> **- Mark 9:23 (KJV)**

Three-Time Survivor, Forever Faithful

As a three-time breast cancer survivor, I have always kept my faith in God. Keep your faith in God, be your own advocate every step of the way, and keep on surviving and thriving. We have to keep fighting.

Because of the tumor disappearing, I will have to have CT scans every 3 to 6 months, and I'm okay with that. At this point, I've had four CT scans, and there's no evidence of anything but God.

I continue every three weeks to get my treatment of Herceptin, and I'm doing very well. I get an echo of my heart every four months, and my heart is doing good—no damage from the medication. My oncologist would love to keep me on this medication indefinitely, but you never know what God's plans are.

My Message to You

I want to encourage you to listen to your body and be your own advocate. When they tell you, "Oh, it's nothing," but you know it's something, we all as women know we need a mammogram every year. Make sure you get that.

Remember to keep your faith. Stay strong. We have the strength to get through anything. My favorite verse is "I can do all things through Christ that strengthens me."

The breast cancer journey is not an easy one. If you feel depressed along your journey, remember there's always someone out there who can help you get through this, but I say keep your faith. God is good.

I must say, as a three-time breast cancer survivor, I learned a lot about myself—how strong and how powerful I can be with God. Nothing is impossible. I walked my journey one day at a time, some days good, some days bad, but I continued to keep my faith, and I kept pressing because there is life after breast cancer.

The saying is: I had cancer, but cancer did not have me.

So, whenever you're feeling down, give it to God, and He will handle everything. Everything in life is one day at a time.

God is good, and there is power in faith, prayer, and believing that miracles still happen today.

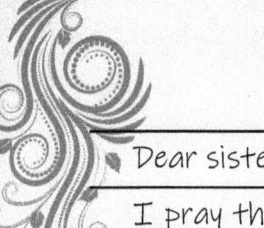

Dear sister,

I pray that this finds you well and in good spirits. The one thing that I want you to remember is that God Loves you, He always has, and He always will and that He is Good and He is Faithful. I had to learn this for myself with the help of the Holy Spirit of Course. Because sometimes our perspective of God can be off, especially when we are going through something that we never expected and fear creeps in like a thief in the night and we are devastated. Going through so many different emotions and the enemy is constantly whispering lies that this thing here is going to take us out but even though it may not look like it or feel like know that He is who He says He is and that He is with you even if you cannot see Him, feel Him, or hear Him, He is there and that He promises to never leave you nor forsake you. He never has and he never will. Remember when Jesus told the disciples to get in the boat and cross over to the other side and in the middle of them getting to the other side a storm came and they were afraid and Jesus was asleep in the boat and they asked Him if he cared that they perish (He did). Jesus got up, and said to the storm Peace be still and despite the storm they ended up on the other side. Then when Jesus told Peter to come to him on the water and when Peter was going to Jesus a storm rose and Peter took his eyes off Jesus and he began to sink and He asked Jesus to save him (He did) and Jesus reached down and pulled him out of the water and they walked back to the boat together. See when trouble or storms come and we stay focused on the storms and we focus on the storms instead of Jesus and we don't praise, worship, and keep our focus on what He promised we begin to sink under the pressures in our lives but no matter the storm, no matter what your storm is whether it be breast cancer, sickness, finances, your children, or your marriage with Jesus on your boat He will get you on the other side of whatever your facing. Be encouraged my sister and know without a shadow of a doubt that with Jesus we are going to get to the other side of whatever you're this is. I pray that you be blessed and encouraged by this entire book and my chapter. I love you but God loves you best!!!

Valerie

He Did it For Me!
Overcoming Cancer with Jesus

Authored By: Valerie Wilder

I was lying in bed one evening when I heard it clear as day: "Breast Cancer." My immediate response was what we all say first: "The devil is a liar!" I rebuked it, got up, put on my clothes, and went about my days and life as usual. I had no idea that the Holy Spirit was warning me about what was to come. Sometimes God's voice comes to prepare us, not to scare us, but I wasn't ready to receive that truth yet.

One early Sunday morning in June 2007, I went to church, and my Pastor, Pastor Karol Warren, prophesied to me: "God is healing you from something."

I said, "Lord, I thank You in advance for healing me from whatever it is."

Little did I know that the "whatever it is" was already growing inside my body, and God was already orchestrating my healing journey.

When God Closes Doors to Open Windows

In July 2007, I started a daycare because I had gotten laid off from my job at Portsmouth Naval Hospital after the contract ended. I had five children in my daycare, and I loved caring for my babies. These weren't just clients to me—they were precious souls I got to nurture every day.

But in August 2007, three of my parents took their children out of my daycare and put them in regular school. Now I only had my two grandsons to care for. I was confused and hurt. "What is going on? Am I doing something wrong?"

Then my daughter came with news that broke my heart: "Mom, I have decided to put the boys in regular school too."

I was blown away. The feeling that I was not as good of a daycare provider as I thought haunted me. I went over a checklist multiple times to make sure I had done all the things I should have done as a daycare provider. I made sure my babies were fed, clean, educated, and loved. I even made sure they were prepared for bed when they left me—I bathed them, and they smelled so good when they went home.

I did not understand what was happening. Unbeknownst to me, my journey with cancer had already begun, and God was clearing my schedule for what was ahead.

Every day, my son would call me with the same question: "Ma, have you been looking for a job yet?"

"No, I don't want to go to work outside of my home," I would tell him.

He kept calling me every day. "Have you looked in the newspaper? You need to cut out at least ten jobs from the paper and apply."

I got so tired of him calling me that I finally gave up and said, "Ok! I'm going to apply."

So I started looking for a job. I went to a place called Opportunity Inc. and applied for a position at Eastern Virginia Medical School. I got hired in August 2007. Praise God, I was working, although I did not want to work outside my home. Looking back, I can see God's hand moving even in my resistance.

Divine Insurance

When I went for orientation, they offered us health insurance, and my first down payment would be $500 out of my first check. I went home and talked to my husband about it, and we agreed it was not a good time. I was not sick or anything—at least I thought—and we decided to wait until the next enrollment month because we were behind on bills and needed the money.

So I told Human Resources that I was not going to get the health insurance.

Later that week, a lady from Human Resources called me and asked if the reason I was not getting health insurance was because of financial reasons. I said yes.

She said, "My supervisor told me to tell you that we are not going to take $500 out of your first check but $150 so that you can get your insurance."

I was so grateful, not realizing that a month later I was going to desperately need this insurance. God already knew what I was going to need and made the way before I even knew I needed a way.

The Examination I Never Planned

At the end of August, I was taking a shower, and afterward, I lay down on my bed. What happened next was not my idea—it was as if the Holy Spirit Himself led me to do a breast exam.

Now, unfortunately, I did not do regular breast exams, but it was as if He laid me down, took my hand, and guided me. He didn't say, "Valerie, do a breast exam." It was supernatural guidance that I can't fully explain.

On my right breast, I felt something that felt pea-sized. I asked my husband to check it, and he felt the same thing. Strangely, I never checked my left breast because I was so concerned about what I'd found on the right.

The next day, I called and made an appointment with my primary care physician, Dr. Charlene Robertson, and got an appointment for September 1st.

She did a breast exam, feeling the right breast first, and then she felt the left. Suddenly, she stopped.

"Mrs. Wilder, I feel something over here on your left side and nothing on the right side," she said. "It feels like the size of a golf ball. I am going to make you an appointment with Dr. Jennifer Reed to have them do a biopsy."

A golf ball. The thing I felt was pea-sized, but the real problem was something I hadn't even noticed. God had led me to discover what I could feel so that doctors could find what I couldn't feel.

The Peace That Passes Understanding

On September 17th, I had an appointment with Dr. Jennifer Reed for a biopsy. After the procedure, I went home and returned to work the next day, trying to maintain some normalcy while waiting for results that would change everything.

On September 24th, as I was working, I got the phone call. Dr. Reed informed me that my results came back positive for ductal carcinoma with mucinous features.

I cannot explain the overwhelming peace of God that came over me in that moment. I did not have any panicked feelings then or even after. When I say that God's peace surpasses all understanding, it truly does.

I told my coworkers and my boss, and they were crying, but I was not. I was actually trying to muster up a cry because I thought to myself, "Shouldn't I be crying, torn up from the floor up?" But I wasn't. God had told me through Pastor Warren that He was healing me, and I believed Him. He kept me in His perfect peace when this phone call came.

Dr. Reed asked me to bring my family to the office because she wanted all of them to be told together. I will never forget the look on their faces when she delivered the news. They were truly worried about me. They loved me, and this news was very devastating for them.

My son later told me that when the doctor delivered the news, he was watching me and noticed that I looked so peaceful and unbothered. He said he couldn't cry in that moment because of the calmness he saw in me. However, he shared that afterward, he went into the employee's lounge and broke down—crying, screaming, and throwing furniture.

I prayed that the same peace God gave me in that moment would also be given to my family. You know, they never let their fear show in front of me because they loved me and didn't want to upset me or get me worried. Praise God for my family!

"You will keep in perfect peace those whose minds are steadfast, because they trust in you." Isaiah 26:3 (ESV)

When God Says No

On November 30, 2007, I underwent a mastectomy at Sentara Leigh Hospital in Norfolk, Virginia, performed by Dr. Jennifer Reed with my family by my side.

The night before my surgery, my husband told me something that I initially dismissed: "The Holy Spirit told me that you do not need to get the breast reconstruction."

I said okay, but I went along with the breast reconstruction anyway. Sometimes we hear God clearly but still lean on our own understanding.

An attempted breast reconstruction was conducted by Dr. Theodore Uroskie. I say "attempted" because what happened next proved that Father truly knows best.

During the procedure, Dr. Uroskie pulled skin from my back and placed it on the area where my left breast had been removed. When I was back in my hospital room with my family around me, my daughter came to my bedside, looked at me, and said, "Mom, your face is green."

She pulled back my gown, and the skin on my chest from my back had turned black. There were not enough blood vessels to supply blood to that area, so they had to take me back into the operating room to remove the dead skin.

Praise God for using my daughter to notice my skin color and the area on my chest, because I could have died from the complications. The outcome was a testament that Father knows best. When God says no, even when we don't understand why, His no is protection.

The Reality of Recovery

I was discharged from the hospital on December 1, 2007. The reality of what I was going through hit me most when I was alone, dealing with the practical aspects of recovery that no one prepares you for.

I had to change a surgical drain by myself daily—a thin, flexible rubber tube that was inserted into the area where my breast had been, allowing fluid to flow out to a collection bulb that had to be emptied. Doing this task alone, looking at where my breast used to be, was when the human reality of my situation would settle in.

I realized this was very hard and overwhelming for my family to see me go through, but they prayed, stayed in faith, and continued to support me during this time. They did their best given the circumstances, and I knew they loved me.

I talked to my daughter about how this experience was different from other challenges I'd faced. She said that she had seen me have a certain look in my eyes during past situations and wasn't sure if I was going to make it, but this time when she looked into my eyes, she said, "Okay, we are going to fight." And that is what we did with the Lord on our side.

My daughter and my friend Anne would come and help take care of me and encourage me when they could. I was so grateful for that. It is so good to be with family and friends during our trying times.

Sometimes I did feel sad, but God helped me get over that. I could not let my emotions take control over me and carry me down a depressed and lonely path. God was with me, and I realized that in times when I felt alone, I wasn't really alone, because He was always there.

I thank God for the strength and peace He gave me to still be able to do the things I used to do at home, even while healing from major surgery.

Walking Through Treatment

After the surgery, I had chemotherapy and twenty-one rounds of radiation. I thank God that I was able to work throughout my treatment, which was not something I took for granted.

People told me that I would get sick from the chemo and burned from the radiation, but neither of those things happened to me. My labs remained normal throughout treatment. Praise God, because when you are on chemotherapy, it kills every good and bad cell in your body, but somehow God preserved my strength.

I remember when my hair fell out. My husband was washing my hair, and all of it started falling out. In an instant, it was gone. But I was so grateful that God blessed me with a daughter who is a cosmetologist. She would style my wigs for me, and I would go to Creative Images to get my bras and prosthetics.

One day, I told my husband I was going to go outside without my wig or a hat and see what people would say. As if I needed to worry about what people would say! But nobody paid me any attention at all.

The day finally came when I was so excited that it was my turn to ring that bell after all twenty-one rounds of radiation were done and the chemotherapy treatments were over. Praise God!

Learning to Live Differently

Learning to live with one breast was an adjustment I hadn't anticipated. Getting dressed became different. Shopping for clothes required new considerations. Simple things like hugging people felt different.

But when I look down at my missing breast, it reminds me that God loves me and that He is so faithful. Could He have healed me from cancer without surgery? Of course. Sometimes doubt, fear, or other things can get in the way of us receiving the manifestation of God's divine healing, but God is faithful. Every good and perfect gift comes from Him, so He will use doctors and technology to do things like mastectomies to heal us—He created them anyway.

He even made a prosthetic just for me to put in my bra. He loves me, and He was with me through it all. In the midst of it all, He kept me, and He was carrying me in His arms through everything.

More Than a Survivor

All the glory and the victory belong to Jesus because He overcame the cancer that was in my body so that it would not overtake me. Jesus reminds us in John 16:33 that in this world we will have trouble, but we should be of good cheer because He has overcome the world, and He will NEVER leave us nor forsake us.

I am an overcomer, not just a survivor, because Jesus overcame cancer and everything that the enemy tried to bring my way. God is faithful, and I cannot say that enough. I am grateful for the love He has for me. He is my Heavenly Father and knows what is best for me, whether it be a miracle or a mastectomy. He worked it all out for my good, ahead of time.

Now I can tell His story to the world and let everyone know that He did it for me, and He will do the same for you. Trust and believe. He will take care of you in your storm. You are never alone. He rescued me, and He will rescue you.

"The Lord your God goes with you; he will never leave you nor forsake you." Deuteronomy 31:8 (ESV)

Living the Testimony

Today, years later, I live as a walking testimony of God's faithfulness. When women ask me about my experience, I tell them that it wasn't just about surviving cancer—it was about discovering how deeply God loves us even in our most frightening moments.

I share how God prepared everything I needed before I even knew I needed it: the job with insurance, the peace that sustained me, the family support, even the warning that allowed me to be somewhat prepared for what was coming.

I've learned that being an overcomer means more than just getting through something difficult. It means allowing God to use your experience to help others see His faithfulness. It means trusting His plan even when it includes suffering. It means finding joy and purpose in the midst of circumstances you never would have chosen.

I am so grateful for my family and friends who stood by my side, who prayed for me, and cared for me whether near or far. Thank You, Jesus—You did it for me!

I pray that my testimony of how God brought me through my journey with breast cancer encourages you. As my sister in Christ, Trina Luster, said: "It was not the end but the beginning of my treatment."

"And we know that in all things God works for the good of those who love him, who have been called according to his purpose." Romans 8:28 (ESV)

If you are walking through your own storm right now, remember that you are not alone. The same God who carried me will carry you. The same peace that sustained me is available to you. The same faithfulness I experienced is yours to claim.

Trust Him. He knows what He's doing, even when you don't understand. He is working everything out for your good, even when it doesn't feel good. And He will never, ever leave you to face anything alone.

You are an overcomer. Not because you're strong enough, but because He is.

Dear Sister,

I am sharing my story with you because my God is Jehovah Rafa (the God that heals us) and He is no respecter of person, He did it for me and He'll do the same for you. I pray that you are blessed by my story.

                                              Via

Victory is Mine!
Authored By: Via May-Shephard

*"When thou passest through the waters,
I will be with thee; and through the rivers, they shall not
overflow thee: when thou walkest through the fire, thou shalt
not be burned; neither shall the flame kindle upon thee."*
Isaiah 43:2

In March 2010, a few days before or just after my 56th birthday, I returned to the hospital for a follow-up mammogram. I've been getting mammograms since I was 35 years old. My aunt and great-aunt both had breast cancer diagnoses and double mastectomies. My breasts are dense, so it was not at all unusual for the radiologist to want more pictures or an ultrasound.

Yet something inside me whispered "this is different" as I walked up to the mammogram machine.

That whisper. I can't explain it, but it was distinct from my usual pre-mammogram anxiety. This felt like a divine nudge, preparing me for something I wasn't ready to face. You know how sometimes God prepares our hearts before He reveals what's ahead? That's what this felt like. It wasn't audible, but it was unmistakable—like someone had just told me my life was about to change forever, and deep down, I already knew it was true.

After reading the new X-rays, the technician confirmed that they saw a suspicious mass and they wanted to do a biopsy as soon as possible. In fact, they had an opening that morning and I agreed to have the procedure done.

I was there alone—routine visit, I thought—and terrified of being awake for a biopsy. Because I was alone, they couldn't put me to sleep, so it was do it now or come back later. I'm the world's biggest chicken, but I had to know as soon as possible.

The procedure was terribly invasive and painful for me. An unsuspecting nurse offered to hold my right hand throughout the procedure. She had no idea what she was signing up for! I pray that her hand and fingers recovered without injury.

Looking back, I realize that going alone to what I thought was a routine appointment was actually part of God's plan. He knew I needed to face this first moment of truth by myself, to lean completely on Him before bringing my support system into the battle.

The Wrestling Season

After the biopsy, you wait for what seems like forever—days—for the results. I prayed as I waited and asked the intercessors at my church to lift me up daily in prayer.

My greatest fear was not death. I firmly believed that God had bigger plans for me and that my assignment wasn't finished. I didn't even doubt that God could bring me through it if it turned out to be malignant. I simply did not want to go through it.

The very thought of chemotherapy and its impacts on the body terrified me. I'd lose my hair, I sobbed. VANITY at its best! Here I was, a 56-year-old woman more worried about my hair than my life. But you know what? I've learned that God meets us in our vanity just as much as He meets us in our nobility. He didn't shame me for crying over my hair—He understood that sometimes our deepest fears show up in the most unexpected ways.

Those waiting days became a wrestling match with God that I didn't know I needed. One minute I was pacing my kitchen declaring, "By His stripes I am healed!" and the next minute I was curled up on my bathroom floor sobbing, "God, I can't do this." I discovered that having faith doesn't mean you don't feel fear—it means you choose to trust God even when fear is screaming so loud you can barely hear His voice.

The Moment Everything Shifted

Within a few days, my doctor—who was also a personal friend and sister in Christ—called me late one evening with the results of the biopsy. She asked if my husband Stan was home and asked me to have him join the call, which turned out to be life-changing news.

The moment she asked for Stan, I knew. You don't ask for the husband to be on the call for good news.

I felt like I was having an out-of-body experience. I was so quiet that Dr. Norwood asked if I was still in the room. I was numb and in shock. How could God allow this to happen to me? He knows that I'm a chicken and He's supposed to love me. He did then and He loves me still, yet I asked, "Why me?"

The "why me?" question consumed me for weeks. I threw it at God during sleepless nights, whispered it through tears while folding laundry, and screamed it in my car when I was alone. I felt betrayed, abandoned, and confused. Here I was, serving God, raising babies, trying to live right, and this is what I get?

But somewhere in the middle of one of those crying sessions—I can't even tell you exactly when—the question shifted. Maybe it was when I saw a mother at the grocery store with her sick child, or maybe it was during a particularly honest conversation with God, but suddenly I wasn't asking "Why me?" anymore.

I was asking, "Why not me?"

Why should I be exempt from the struggles that touch so many other women? What made me so special that I should sail through life without facing the battles that refine us, strengthen us, and ultimately reveal God's power in ways we never knew we needed? That shift didn't happen because I got super spiritual overnight. It happened because I finally stopped demanding that God explain Himself and started asking Him to use whatever He allowed for His glory and my good.

Love Finds a Way

At the time of my diagnosis, my husband and I had two young children—a four-year-old son and a seven-month-old daughter. The children I'd prayed for all of my life. I was gripped by fear.

How would I take care of my babies? Would my son be traumatized seeing his mother in pain with tubes hanging from the area where her breast once was? My children are adopted, and my daughter's adoption had not yet been finalized. She was still legally placed with us in foster care, but we'd had her since the day she was born.

The "what ifs" quickly set in. What if they take her from me because I'm unable to care for her right now? After all, I was a 56-year-old woman with two children under the age of five who was now a 56-year-old woman with breast cancer!

The fear of losing my daughter through the adoption system felt almost as terrifying as the cancer diagnosis itself. Here I was, fighting for my life while simultaneously fighting to keep my family together. The timing felt cruel—just as we were on the verge of making our family official, cancer threatened to tear it apart.

To add to my despair, I was further devastated when the doctor said I wouldn't be able to lift anything over five pounds. That meant I couldn't pick up my daughter or my son for months. How could I possibly not pick up my beautiful babies?

I remember the first day after surgery when my son ran to me with his arms outstretched, expecting his usual pick-up-and-swing-around greeting. The look of confusion on his face when I couldn't lift him nearly broke me. "Mama's hurt right now, baby," I managed to say, but how do you explain cancer to a four-year-old?

My husband, in all his faith, love, and wisdom, reminded me that the doctor didn't say I couldn't hold them. So during my recovery, he would place a pillow on my chest as a barrier and lay our daughter on the pillow so that I could hold her and spend time with her. Those moments became sacred to me—her tiny body rising and falling with my breathing, her complete trust that Mama was still Mama even with tubes and bandages and all the medical equipment.

My son learned to crawl up beside me on the couch, careful not to bump my chest, and we'd read books together with his head on my shoulder. Cancer tried to steal my ability to physically comfort my children, but love found a way. Stan's creativity in helping me maintain that connection with our babies was one of the most beautiful expressions of love I've ever experienced. It showed me that when life throws limitations at love, love gets creative.

"He heals the brokenhearted and binds up their wounds."
Psalm 147:3 (ESV)

Surgery Day Realities

A few weeks later, I showed up for my outpatient surgery. I remember thinking, how do they cut your boob halfway off (lumpectomy) and send you home the same day? Yet they did, with two external drains that I wore around my waist in a fanny pack, no pain pump, and instructions for my husband to log the amount in each of the drains and to empty them as frequently as necessary.

Let me tell you, those drains were no joke. Fashion became a secondary concern when you're wearing medical equipment around your waist. I had to learn to dress around drains, sleep with drains, and maintain some dignity while my husband emptied fluid from tubes hanging out of my body.

The nurse who took care of me before my surgery was a breast cancer survivor. I recall her saying to me, "You can do this. It'll be a yucky year post-op, but after that, you'll find your new normal." No truer words were ever spoken.

That nurse became an angel to me in that moment. She didn't sugarcoat the journey ahead, but she gave me hope that there was life on the other side of "yucky." Sometimes that's exactly what we need—not false optimism, but realistic hope from someone who's walked the path ahead of us.

When One Became Three

At my post-op visit, I learned that there were not one, but three tumors hiding in there, and I was diagnosed with Stage 2 breast cancer. The doctor also shared that they had not cleared the margins and that additional surgery would be necessary. The good news was that the cancer had not spread to my lymph nodes.

Three tumors. THREE.

When you think you're dealing with one problem and discover there are actually three, it feels like life is playing a cruel joke. But I've learned that God sometimes allows us to see challenges one layer at a time because we couldn't handle seeing it all at once. If I had known from the beginning that I had three tumors, would I have had the courage to even start this fight?

Surgery number two of many that year resulted in removing the left breast (mastectomy) and reconstructive surgery to place the implant. I was in surgery four to six hours that day, and my husband and I even got to stay overnight!

Before the second procedure, the doctor asked us to consider a double mastectomy. Doing so would give me two new breasts, and since I wasn't blessed with much cleavage or bust, the option was somewhat appealing to me. Not only would new boobs get me off the itty-bitty-titty committee and give me the bust I'd always dreamed of, it would also reduce the risk of cancer showing up in the right breast in the future.

Though very tempting, we decided against the double mastectomy and my only opportunity to ditch the B-cup! While I've questioned that decision a few times over the years—especially when the doctors found a mass in my right breast that thankfully was benign—I am very grateful for my one little boob.

Looking back, I realize I was trying to find humor in a situation that felt overwhelming. Sometimes laughter is the only way to cope with decisions about your body that you never imagined having to make. The fact that I could joke about cup sizes while facing a mastectomy shows how the human spirit adapts to protect itself.

The Treatment Decision

After the second surgical procedure, my breast tissue was sent to a lab in California for a test called Oncotype DX. The test results would help my doctors decide if chemotherapy along with hormone therapy would lower the risk of cancer recurrence. The results take several weeks, and the decision on chemotherapy for me was directly tied to the results of this test.

Again, we prayed as we waited. This waiting period felt different from the first one. Now I knew what we were dealing with, but I still didn't know what treatment would be required. The uncertainty was almost worse than the initial diagnosis.

During those weeks of waiting, I found myself having the most honest conversations with God I'd ever had in my life. I told Him about my fears of chemotherapy, my concerns about my children seeing me sick, my worry about the adoption finalization. I laid it all out before Him like never before, and in that raw honesty, I felt closer to Him than I ever had.

Oncotype test results present as a score from 0-100. A score of 25 or less indicates a lower risk of cancer recurrence, and chemotherapy is not believed to be beneficial because the side effects outweigh its benefits. A score of 26 or higher indicates a high risk of recurrence, and chemotherapy is strongly recommended.

My score came in at 25—right on the threshold. My oncologist recommended that I take chemotherapy, but he left the decision to my husband and me. Chemo or not?

That would be a NO for me!

This wasn't a decision I made lightly or flippantly. I spent hours researching, praying, and weighing the risks and benefits with Stan. Being right at the threshold meant the medical community was essentially saying, "We're not sure if this will help you or harm you more." In that uncertainty, I chose to trust my gut and my God rather than subject my body to treatment that might not provide significant benefit.

Some people questioned my decision. Some thought I was being foolish or reckless. But when you're facing treatment decisions, you have to live with the consequences of your choice. I chose the path that felt right for my body, my family situation, and my faith journey.

The Daily Commitment

I did agree to take Tamoxifen for the next five years. Tamoxifen is a hormone therapy drug used to decrease the risk of cancer returning. I am not a pill popper and I don't like shots, so this became another difficult decision point for me.

Could I actually put this medication in my body every day for the next five years? The jury was still out on the side effects of hormone therapy, and I was no more interested in this medication than I was the chemotherapy. What if we created another issue? What if, what if?

I did commit to taking this pill daily, and God blessed me to not experience any of the side effects that can go along with this regimen. Every morning for five years, I swallowed that little white pill and trusted God to protect my body from both cancer recurrence and medication side effects.

That daily pill became a symbol of my commitment to fighting for my life while trusting God with the outcome. Some days I took it with gratitude, other days with reluctance, but I took it faithfully because I had made a promise to myself and my family to do everything in my power to stay healthy.

My Village of Warriors

I'd like to pay special tribute to my amazing caregivers: my husband Stan Shephard; my sister/friend and rock, Daphne Davis, who was at every appointment, every procedure, and constantly at my bedside; Ronda Lloyd, whose unwavering love, presence, and support strengthened me more than she knows. My daughter Lenora Kennedy-Rhodes helped Papa with the babies. Elder Callie Wright, who has gone on to be with the Lord, bombarded heaven on my behalf. My mom, Helen E. May, who stepped into eternity last year, and First Lady Gwen Cast (who I am honored to serve and call my friend), was always there for me and with me.

Each of these people played a crucial role in my survival, but more than that, they showed me what the body of Christ looks like in action.

Daphne never missed an appointment—not one. She sat through every consultation, held my hand during procedures, and celebrated small victories with me. When I was too nervous to ask the doctor questions, she asked them for me. When I couldn't remember what the doctor said because I was overwhelmed, she took notes. That kind of faithful friendship is rare and precious.

Stan didn't just care for me; he became the primary caregiver for our small children while working full-time and managing my medical needs. He never complained, never made me feel like a burden, never suggested that this was more than he signed up for. He loved me through cancer the same way he loved me through health—completely and unconditionally. When I felt like damaged goods, he treated me like a treasure.

Elder Wright's prayers were like a spiritual covering over our entire family. She would call just to pray with me over the phone, sometimes for thirty minutes or more. Her faith was contagious and strengthening. When my faith felt weak, I could lean on hers.

My mother's love and worry were palpable. She couldn't take the cancer away, but she could love me through it, and she did with every phone call, every visit, every expression of concern. Sometimes a mother's love is the most healing medicine there is.

First Lady Cast's friendship was like a warm blanket during the coldest parts of my journey. She had a way of making me feel normal when everything else about my life felt abnormal. Her "pats" are therapeutic.

> *"As iron sharpens iron, so one person sharpens another."*
> **Proverbs 27:17 (ESV)**

Fourteen Years of Victory

So here we are in 2024—fourteen years later. I am a survivor and I am cancer-free! I've lost a few friends along the way to the disease that I miss terribly: Shaunda, Joe, and Penny.

Someone said to me once, "Is your cancer in remission?" Satan, get thee behind me! I said to them, "I plead the blood of Jesus against that buffoonery. I am not in remission; I am cancer-free; and I am healed in Jesus' great name." #viajussayin

That distinction matters to me. Remission implies that cancer is still lurking, waiting to return. Healing implies that God has completely restored my body. I choose to stand on healing rather than remission because my faith is in a God who doesn't do halfway measures.

I learned a lot about life and myself on this journey. Life is precious—never take it for granted. We are not confident of the rest of this day, let alone tomorrow. I love hard and tell my family, friends, and others in my circle that I love them often. I cherish life more than ever, and I'm so grateful for every day that I get to spend with those that I love so dearly.

Cancer taught me to live with an urgency that I didn't have before. Not a frantic urgency, but a purposeful one. Every conversation matters. Every hug counts. Every moment is a gift.

My walk with God has never been the same. I now know Him as healer for myself. No one can tell me anything different or take that away from me. I trusted and depended on Him to bring me through and to take care of my husband and children while He did so. I'm here to tell you that He is faithful.

Before cancer, I knew God intellectually as a healer—I had read about it, heard testimonies about it, believed in it theoretically. After cancer, I know God experientially as MY healer. There's a difference between knowing about God's power and experiencing God's power personally. One is head knowledge; the other is heart transformation.

Walking in Victory

I have had the opportunity to share my testimony with other women affected by this disease who are on the battlefield. I am humbled that God would use me to encourage someone else.

When I share my story, I'm always careful to emphasize that my journey is uniquely mine. I don't encourage women to skip chemotherapy or make the same treatment decisions I made. What I do encourage them to do is pray, research, get multiple opinions, and make decisions that align with their faith, their medical situation, and their personal circumstances.

Every woman's cancer journey is different, but every woman deserves to know that she's not fighting alone. Whether she chooses chemotherapy or doesn't, whether she has surgery or doesn't, whether she pursues traditional treatment or alternative treatment, she deserves support and encouragement.

My victory isn't just about surviving cancer—it's about learning to trust God with outcomes I can't control. It's about discovering that love shows up in hospital rooms and uncomfortable conversations. It's about finding out that I'm stronger than I thought but also more fragile than I pretended to be.

The adoption of our daughter was finalized while I was in treatment. The social worker saw a family fighting to stay together rather than a woman too sick to care for a child. Sometimes what we think will disqualify us actually demonstrates our qualification in ways we never expected.

My children don't remember their mother as a sick person. They remember her as someone who fought hard to be present for them, who found creative ways to show love even when physically limited, who never let cancer steal their sense of security or their belief that Mama was invincible.

"And we know that in all things God works for the good of those who love him, who have been called according to his purpose."
Romans 8:28 (ESV)

To My Sister Walking This Path

I pray that my story has in some way touched and enriched your life. Be encouraged, my sister—we serve a great big God, and He does more than we can even think or imagine. Cancer is no match for my God. #viajussayin

If you're facing a cancer diagnosis, know that your journey will be uniquely yours. Don't compare your path to mine or anyone else's. Trust God to guide you through your specific circumstances with your specific needs in mind.

If you're a caregiver, know that your presence matters more than your words. Sometimes just showing up is the most powerful thing you can do.

If you're a survivor, know that your testimony has power. Share it when you can, even if it's just with one person who needs to hear that victory is possible.

Victory doesn't always look like we expect it to. Sometimes victory is choosing treatment, sometimes it's choosing not to. Sometimes victory is complete physical healing, sometimes it's peace in the midst of ongoing struggle. But victory is always available when we trust God with our outcomes.

My God is Jehovah Rapha—the God who heals. He healed my body, but He also healed my perspective, my priorities, and my purpose. He can do the same for you.

Cancer tried to write my ending, but God had the final word. And His word over your life is victory, too.

Embracing Change

By Tara Tucker

Wednesday, December 14, 2016 – Journal Entry

"I must be very strong, because a lot keeps happening in my life—yet God says He will never put more on me than I can handle. So I have to be strong and handle it all.

I lost my mom and got cancer in the same year. But in that same year, I also got a salon and celebrated my first year as a homeowner. It's weird. Emotions. Joy and pain... anger and sadness. I'm currently sitting in confusion and shock. I seem okay outwardly, but inwardly, I am not. It's been six days since I received the news, and I'm still trying to process it all. Today, that processing involved a tall glass of wine—and then some. That isn't normal behavior for me and hasn't been in years, but today, I truly felt overwhelmed.

I remember when I got the call. I was waiting for my next—and last—client of the day. It was 3 PM on Thursday, December 8, 2016. Dr. McCarthy called and said she had bad news. Somehow, in the back of my mind, I already knew. I had felt it during the ultrasound and biopsy. When she asked if it was okay to talk on the phone, I said yes. I was not about to wait and come into the office—oh no.

So she told me: invasive ductal carcinoma. Wow.

She reassured me it was in the early stages and went over the pathology report. She mentioned a surgeon and explained a few other things. I was writing down what she was saying, but it all felt like a blur. I was in a daze, if that makes sense. I hung up the phone, and that's when I realized—I was shaking.

"Well, okay, God," I said. "Here we go."

Reading these words now, years later, I can still feel the weight of that moment. The year 2016 was supposed to be a year of celebration and new beginnings. I had just bought my first home, opened my storefront salon, and was finally stepping into the life I'd dreamed of creating. But in the same year, I lost my mother suddenly to a heart attack, and then I received a cancer diagnosis.

Oh, the highs and lows of life.

Looking back, I realize losing my mother prepared me in ways I couldn't understand at the time. Seeing her after her transition—lying on her side in her bed, facing the television, the remote still in her hand—taught me something about the fragility of life. About how quickly everything can change.

One day, she was here; the next, she was gone.

One day, I was cancer-free; the next, I was preparing for a double mastectomy.

The Discovery That Changed My Path

It started with a simple thought during my shower at the end of September 2016. Out of the blue, I had this inner prompting: *Do a self-breast exam.* I had never been diligent about self-exams, but something made me pause and listen to that inner voice.

Now I know—it was the Holy Spirit prompting me.

I raised my left arm and examined my breast, slowly applying a little pressure. Everything felt normal. Then I raised my right arm and repeated the technique… and paused.

This doesn't feel right, I thought. There was a lump on my right breast near my armpit. It felt hard, about the size of a marble.

I froze. *Lord, no. Please, no.*

I got out of the shower, knowing I needed to see my doctor right away. I scheduled an exam with my gynecologist, who saw me immediately and confirmed there was indeed a knot that concerned her. She gave me a referral for a mammogram—my very first.

But fear took over.

I sat on that referral until after my birthday in November. I didn't want to deal with it. I just wanted to enjoy my 40th birthday. I didn't mention my fears to anyone. I kept it inside, hoping—foolishly—that ignoring it would somehow make it go away.

I remember sitting at my birthday dinner in a state of duality—laughing and talking, while internally wondering if I would live to see another birthday. These are the thoughts that enter your mind when you're facing cancer and all that comes with it.

When Everything Falls Apart

Let me take you back to that day. I received the cancer diagnosis while working in my salon. I was in shock, but I kept going. I finished out my clients without saying a word. I laughed, I talked—but my mind was racing, replaying the conversation over and over. When the salon was clean and empty, I locked up and drove home.

There was no music playing. Just silence. I drove slowly, knowing that once I walked through my front door, I would have to share news that would change everything for my family.

I walked into the house, put my purse and coat away, and went into the bathroom. "Help me, Lord," I prayed. I even cooked dinner before I finally sat down with my husband.

He was in his man cave, playing the game. He looked up when I walked in.

"Baby, the doctor called me," I said.

He stopped playing and looked at me closely. "What did she say?"

"That I have breast cancer."

He immediately started crying and held me so tightly. I burst out crying in his arms. It was a sad, but absolutely beautiful, moment. There was an intimacy in it that we might not have ever experienced before. I had been carrying this alone—but now I could finally release it. It felt like a weight had been lifted.

That moment taught me something crucial: we think we're protecting others by keeping our fears to ourselves, but we're actually robbing them of the opportunity to support us—and robbing ourselves of the strength that comes from shared love.

It's wild. My mom hid her heart disease from us. And I was holding my cancer diagnosis, and even the fear that I might have it, when I felt the lump, just as close to the chest.

But what a relief it was to finally say it out loud.

After we cried, we talked about what it would look like moving forward.

The day before surgery, my sister in Christ took my daughters to her home so my husband and I could spend one last night together before our lives changed forever.

Initially, they said it was stage 2. But after surgery, it was determined to be stage 3B. On my son's birthday—January 18, 2017—I had three surgeries: a double mastectomy, a lymph node dissection, and the placement of tissue expanders. It lasted over nine hours.

I had such a huge turnout in the waiting room. The support was overwhelming and beautiful. Support matters. Community matters.

Doctors removed 9 out of 12 infected lymph nodes from under my arm, which led to lymphedema—an extremely painful condition that makes my right arm swell and my hand look like a mitten. It's something I've lived with for the better part of eight years. It's also tried to kill me three times—via cellulitis and sepsis.

When I finally saw my chest, I looked down and saw two small mounds where my breasts used to be. I had always been generous in that area, so this was… jarring. They didn't feel like mine. Tubes hung from my body. I was bruised and sore. I could barely move. I couldn't even lift my arms over my head.

The doctors and nurses kept talking about my "new normal," and I was just trying to wrap my head around what that even meant.

Many people still had no idea I even had cancer—let alone that I was undergoing a double mastectomy. But the Lord led me to open up. He told me that my journey would help others. That made me uncomfortable, but I was obedient. I began writing and sharing my testimony.

In the days and weeks following surgery, God would not allow everyone to be around me. Certain people were placed in my life to pour into me spiritually—and I thank God for them. So many from my church stepped up to bring meals and check on me. My husband and I were deeply touched by their care and concern.

Then came more revelations.

Tests showed I had BRCA2—a mutated, cancer-causing gene. Because of the high risk of ovarian cancer, my doctor suggested I have my ovaries removed within the next year or two. I nodded as I received piece after piece of news. So many doctors, so many professionals. It was overwhelming.

I wanted to scream, *Geez, leave my body alone!*

But I didn't scream. I did what so many women do—I held it together on the outside while falling apart on the inside.

The Season of Silence

It was Christmas, and I didn't want to ruin it for my children. So I kept quiet. I watched my children open their gifts and silently wondered if I would be there the following Christmas. The fear was real. And it was overwhelming.

By that time, I had finally confided in a select few; those I knew were prayer warriors and would actually pray for me.

But I didn't tell my kids—until just days before surgery.

I kept rehearsing what I would say. I kept wondering when the right moment would come. Time was running out. I met with each of them individually.

My youngest daughter looked at me, wide-eyed, and asked, "Mommy, are you going to die?"

"No, baby. I'm not going to die."

That was enough for her. After that, she just took care of me in her own little way—just like she did when her grandmother passed.

Talk about a reality check.

My life was not in my hands.

What could I do?

My older daughter and son were shocked, scared, and sad. Each of my children responded with love and support.

In those moments, nothing else mattered. Not work. Not my hair. Not even the cancer itself. Just God and my family. I thought about life. I wondered what its quality would be like going forward. I wondered who I would become. I worried—would I survive? Would this change my marriage? Would I still be me?

My prayer was: *Lord, take this away from me. Give me that miraculous healing—the one where the tumor disappears before the next scan.*

My sister Angela prayed the same.

It was such an emotionally difficult time. My sisters in Christ prayed with me and encouraged me. And then, I received a word from the Lord: *This will not be unto death. Be encouraged.*

I wanted more details. I wanted Him to say something else—anything. But I held on to that one promise. I wanted the testimony of being healed *without* surgery and treatment, but that wasn't my story.

I had to go *through* it.

And now, looking back, I understand: sometimes healing doesn't come by avoiding the process. Sometimes, the miracle *is* the process—and the strength and transformation that come with it.

I was never the same again.

There was the woman before cancer. And there was the one after.

The Loneliness of Being Strong

As more people found out, they started calling, texting, and offering advice: "Take chemo," "Don't take chemo," "Eat this way," "Try this supplement." Everyone had something to say. And of course, "Don't worry—God's got you."

Easy to say.

Yes, I knew God had me. But I still worried. I still feared. They didn't have cancer. They didn't know what was happening inside my mind and body. So despite all the love around me, I felt completely alone.

This is something I want other women to understand: it's okay to feel alone even when you're surrounded by people who care. Cancer is an isolating experience because it's happening *inside* of you. Unless someone has walked that exact path, they can't fully understand.

The well-meaning encouragement, the pressure to "stay positive," the suggestions—it all became overwhelming. I wasn't trying to be brave. I was just trying to survive.

I scoured the internet for stories of women in my shoes. Finding them was like finding water in a desert. I joined groups and message boards. I needed understanding. I needed to make sense of what was happening in my body. I was 40 years old, yet I felt like an elderly woman—aching all over, mentally exhausted, and anxious.

From the moment of my diagnosis, through the surgeries and chemo, I had insomnia. I could only sleep with medication. *I would lie awake, night after night, searching for peace, for meaning—anything to make sense of what was happening to me. And in those long, silent hours, I often wished someone had said the right words to me.* That's why I'm sharing my story again—so someone else won't feel as alone as I did. If my words can be that water in a desert for someone else, then it matters. Deeply.

When God Speaks in the Darkness

On January 22, 2017, I heard the Holy Spirit clearly say, "This will be the year of reveals and revelations." I had just come home from the hospital. I didn't fully understand the word at the time, but I wrote it down.

God then told me to prepare a place for Him, and He would meet me there.

We had an extra room in the basement, and I turned it into my prayer room. No shoes allowed—it was holy ground.

After that, my dream life intensified. I also began writing—just as He instructed. I started my *Coffee and Scriptures* blog and began to pour out what I received. Raw. Real. Anointed. Bold. Transparent. That's me.

My writing wasn't clever or cleaned up—it was what it was. I shared prophetic words and allowed the Lord to use me. And over time, I improved—as with any gift you're faithful to steward.

During that time, my ears felt unclogged—like I was hearing Him in a way I never had before. He gave me spiritual eye salve, and suddenly, I could *see*—not just physically, but spiritually. It was like I was seeing for the first time at 40.

While chemotherapy was attacking my body, God was awakening my spirit. He was revealing truths about my identity, my calling, and my relationship with Him.

The Battle

The first surgery was the implanting of the chemo port—a small device under the skin in my chest. It connected to a vein and allowed the nurses to deliver chemotherapy and draw blood without repeated needle sticks.

On Monday, I received my first infusion. Nurses wore hazmat gear when they administered the "red devil"—a nickname for the harsh chemo drug. That image alone was haunting. I sat there for hours, the poison entering my body. As soon as it was done, I started feeling nauseous and weak. Tuesday was worse.

That night, while lying in bed, I had a spiritual encounter. An evil spirit came and whispered, "You're going to die."

It tormented me. I was on my third round of chemo.

"You're almost done, baby," my husband encouraged.

I forced a smile. "Yeah," I replied flatly.

I was scheduled for eight rounds of chemo. "Hooray," I said sarcastically. Five more to go. Nothing about it felt celebratory.

The first round had me crawling on my knees, that same voice whispering death over me. But I found my voice and declared, "I will live and not die!"

The nausea was relentless. Certain smells would turn my stomach, just like pregnancy.

The treatment room was filled with reclining chairs. Everyone there was receiving chemo. I spent about five hours there, four days a week, every other week.

I am thankful to be alive. Some people don't survive this.

I clung to God's word to me: *"This is not unto death."*

Okay, Lord.

That season tested everything I thought I knew about faith. It was the first time since salvation that I fought so hard just to believe. And it wouldn't be the last.

What is going on? Who did I offend? What am I reaping?

Those were the thoughts that tormented me.

But through it all—*You're still God. You're still good.*

I had to constantly check my thoughts and refocus on truth.

When my hair started falling out, it was painful. Literally. The follicles ached. I asked my brother in Christ, Elder Hicks, to shave it off. The pain in that area stopped.

But now, I was bald. My eyebrows and lashes were disappearing. I already felt mutilated from the double mastectomy. And the expanders they'd placed were hard and painful—like bricks in my chest.

Where were my soft, beautiful breasts?

Oh yeah… they tried to kill me.

I had trouble sleeping most nights during those months. On some nights, that aggressive voice returned.

"You will die."

"No," I whispered back. "I will live and not die," I told him to go away.

The Word says to submit to God, *resist the devil, and he will flee.*

God gave me another promise I held onto: *"All will be well. This is just a process you have to go through. And I am with you."*

That demon left. But he came back at other times—to mess with my children, to bring division into my home. Especially while I was weak, physically and emotionally.

But God. He is faithful.

He surrounded me with people who interceded for me and kept me encouraged. This spiritual warfare aspect of cancer is something not many talk about. When your body is weak and your emotions are raw, you become a target.

But the same God who heals bodies also protects minds and strengthens spirits.

> *"The Lord your God is with you, the Mighty Warrior who saves. He will take great delight in you; in His love He will no longer rebuke you, but will rejoice over you with singing."*
> —**Zephaniah 3:17 (ESV)**

The Mirror and the Truth

I stood in front of the mirror, peeking at a face I barely recognized. A clean, bald head. No eyebrows. Barely any lashes.

I slowly lowered my eyes to my chest—not to my breasts, but to the foreign material inside of me. I reached out to touch them. They were hard. I couldn't wait to get those expanders out. They felt so far removed, even while being attached to me.

I looked at my scars—radiation burns, discolored skin, surgical incisions. My right arm and hand were swollen; my hand looked like a mitten. There was excess fluid in my stomach, the top of my back, and even one side of my face.

I did not recognize myself.

"Lord… this is heavy. Help me be okay with this," I prayed.

He allowed me to be stripped.

I reflected on the body I used to have and the life I used to live.

Three years after giving the Lord a "Yes" when He called me—and in that time, I lost my mom, lost my daddy, and gained a cancer diagnosis that transformed my body completely.

That moment in the mirror was my rock bottom. But it was also my turning point.

I had to grieve the woman I was before cancer. I had to mourn the body I'd known for 40 years.

I stood there—until I could stare at myself, until I became comfortable enough not to turn away from the mirror.

I leaned in.

This was my current lot. And I gave the Lord another yes.

Then I had to make a choice: Would I spend the rest of my life mourning what was lost? Or would I embrace what remained—and what was possible?

Embracing the New

From that point forward, I began to embrace my newness.

I am alive. I still have an assignment here on Earth. Praise God!

I promised to live—and to exalt Him—for all the days of my life. That became my posture. A posture of gratitude, surrender, and obedience.

I had a newfound passion for living that many around me didn't fully understand. They got the idea, but they didn't grasp that I was *not* the same. There was no going back. There was no "same." Only *new*.

Each day became a gift.

I started singing more. Dancing more. Laughing harder.

Life was good—not because of perfect circumstances, but because I was here to live it. Praise God!

I leaned into my new profession. I was no longer a hairstylist. And no one could've told me that—I would've laughed in their face. I had plans.

VICTORY IS MINE!

But you know the saying, *"Tell God your plans, and He laughs"*? Yeah, He was cracking up—because the trajectory changed quite a bit.

In the stillness of recovery, God began to renew and increase me spiritually. I sat at home reading, writing, blogging, and spending time in His presence like never before. I had never devoted so much time to Him.

The woman cave I had envisioned—complete with an entertainment system and all—became a sacred space. A prayer room. A meeting place with the Lord.

I published several books, and the Lord guided me to start helping others in this area.

Cancer had forced me to slow down. And in that slowing down, I discovered what I had been missing all along: intimacy with God.

But embracing the new came with new challenges.

My libido was affected. The doctors had to keep my estrogen levels low because the cancer I battled fed on estrogen. As a woman, that just didn't sound right. It felt like yet another layer of loss. And in fact, it was. It affected my marriage.

I developed arthritis, muscle spasms, and neuropathy. New bladder issues emerged. But the worst ongoing battle was the lymphedema. I still live with it.

Each time I get a cut on my right arm or hand, I'm at risk of infection. I can go into sepsis in a matter of hours. And each time I recover, I don't start from zero—I start from the *last* episode, and that setback starts a *new* physical issue. It's relentless.

Mentally and physically, it's taxing.

But there's something remarkable I've discovered: the only time I don't feel pain is when I'm working for the Lord. I could be hurting, having chest pains, dealing with shortness of breath, anything—but when I'm ministering, coaching, or building for the Kingdom, something supernatural takes over.

The Lord covers me.

Nothing that happens to me takes Him by surprise. I trust that He will always perfect the things that concern me. I've learned to accept whatever lot He allows.

Surviving survivorship is hard. But acceptance is key.

When you mourn the past, you invite depression. When you worry about the future, you invite anxiety. But when you stay present—when you live in today—you find peace.

Deal with today's portion.

Things can change. But God's grace and mercy are constant. He is consistent and trustworthy.

I understand my assignment now. And when my work here is finished, I'll go home to be with the Lord.

So I don't worry too much at all. I feel discomfort. I deal with inconvenience. But I'm not tied to this world like that.

I wear it like a loose garment.

Lessons from the Valley

This trial taught me how to be a better person. It stripped me of ego, of control, of certainty—and in that stripping, I found compassion I didn't know I had. I'm more patient now. Softer in some ways, but stronger in others. I see people differently. I listen longer. I forgive faster. Life humbled me—but it also deepened me.

My daughters suffered during this time—not only grieving their grandmother, but also watching their mother fight for her life. They have not been the same. Neither have I.

I'm not the same woman anymore. I keep evolving, and I understand just how short life really is.

I survived something that kills people every day. That awareness changed my whole perspective.

I don't like it when people complain constantly. It's not that I don't understand frustration— I've lived through so much. Believe me, I have things to complain about—LOL.

But honestly? It's just a waste of time.

And I don't like agreeing with the enemy in any way, shape, or form.

Sometimes I mess up and walk by sight. But then I remind myself: *he is a liar,* and God's promises are *yes and amen.* So I repent for any agreement I've made with the enemy—and I change my speech.

I die daily.

I want to love people. I don't want to fight or argue. And if conflict arises, I want it resolved quickly. I'll even apologize when I'm not wrong—just to keep the peace.

I love to laugh. I love to have fun.

I also recognize the sacredness of my circle—the importance of having the *right* people around me. Some people truly meant me no good, no matter how much I loved them. Part of my growth was accepting what people showed me—not what I so desperately wanted to believe.

My parents are gone. Many of my friends have died from the same disease I survived.

I don't care about superficial things anymore. I lean on the Lord for everything.

When you've experienced great loss, your priorities shift.

Permanently.

How could I possibly be the same?

As God continues to take me from faith to faith, I keep shedding old ways of thinking and welcoming new ones. I feel like I'm molting—like an insect shedding its shell and emerging stronger, lighter, more whole.

And I will keep shedding.

I will keep growing.

I will keep expanding.

Even when the enemy whispers fear and doubt, I stand firm. Because I understand who I am—and more importantly, whose I am.

I'm not fighting *for* victory. I'm fighting *from* it.

I don't enter the battle hoping to win. I show up knowing I already have.

But that mindset didn't come easy.

I used to think I loved myself. But I couldn't—not really.

I accepted too much. I shrank too often. I made myself small to make others comfortable.

But not anymore.

Now, I see myself through God's eyes.

Through the loss of my breasts, my hair, and the changes forced on my body, I had to reframe how I saw my beauty and worth. And I do. I love what I see. I am beautifully and wonderfully made.

This body, once used and abused—physically and emotionally—was something I believed was my best asset. I thought my body was what I had to offer. That it was *who* I was. If you read my memoir, *Everybody Kneeling ain't Praying*, then you know what I am referring to.

But I know better now.

God showed me my worth had nothing to do with curves, hair, or external beauty.

And I was blessed with a man who confirmed that truth. He didn't just want my body—he wanted *me*. He saw past the physical and loved my heart, my mind, my spirit.

> *"She is clothed with strength and dignity; s he can laugh at the days to come."*
> **—Proverbs 31:25 (ESV)**

New Boundaries, New Life

I was recently discharged after another long hospital stay battling sepsis.

Another health challenge. Another diagnosis.

Life is short. Life is fragile. We are dust—a vapor.

And just like that, another part of my life changed.

My husband and I are no longer married. It's not what I wanted, but it's what he chose.

After sixteen years together, I now find myself navigating another "new normal"—one I never expected. I wrote about it in an anthology called "SurvivingHer, Unraveled Threads, The Journey of Rebuilding My Life."

It was painful. Another kind of loss. But I've learned that loss has layers. Sometimes it's not just about grieving a person—but grieving the version of life you thought you'd always have.

Still, I move forward.

I still have health challenges, but they don't last forever. They come and go. I adapt.

VICTORY IS MINE!

When I need to sit, I sit. When it's time to move, I move.

People often feel the need to comment on how I move—how I manage so much.

It's funny to me.

God graced me with energy and the ability to multitask. And believe me, when it's time to rest, I do.

But He doesn't ask for permission when He calls someone. So not everyone will understand how He moves in your life.

And that's okay.

No explanation needed.

Just be obedient to the Lord.

I coach women who are called to the marketplace. I help them find their voice, write their books, and position themselves for both impact and income.

This is Kingdom work. And it's time for us to rise up as children of the Most High God.

My priorities have shifted. I no longer allow people to waste my time.

Time is the most precious thing on Earth—and once it's gone, you don't get it back.

People get offended when you set boundaries. Have you noticed that?

Say, "No, today is about me," and some folks act like you've betrayed them.

But I can't let that stop me. I have things to do.

And if saying no—even to family—helps me show up as the woman God called me to be, then so be it.

They understand now.

My children know: Mom needs time to herself.

So she can be good for them—and for the work God assigned her to do.

God and family come first. That wasn't always the case. Often, I chased my bag back in the day.

I've been broken and humbled in many ways.

Seek first His kingdom, and everything else will fall into place.

Cancer taught me that saying no to the wrong things is really saying yes to what matters most.

It taught me that my time and energy are limited—and must be invested wisely.

It taught me that I am not responsible for managing other people's feelings about my boundaries.

Pressure Makes Diamonds

The pain I've experienced… the overwhelming loss… it all propelled me toward my dreams.

I believe in myself—even if no one else does.

Because if God is for me, then it doesn't matter who's against me.

The joy and peace within me now? Indescribable. And no one can take it from me. I can only give it away. And I choose not to.

I believe in God and who He called me to be. He put gifts in me, and now I see myself through the right lens.

I have goals I will accomplish. Pressure makes diamonds.

And baby—I'm sparkling. I'm a jewel.

This is what I want you to understand: cancer may have interrupted your life, but it doesn't have to interrupt your dreams. In fact, it might *clarify* them. *Intensify* them. Give you the courage to chase them like never before.

> *"And we know that in all things God works for the good of those who love Him, who have been called according to His purpose."*
> **—Romans 8:28 (ESV)**

Embracing my "New Normal."

Today, I live as a woman refined by fire.

My body carries scars, yes—but they are evidence of survival. Every mark, every change, tells part of the story: of what I've endured, of what I've overcome, of how God kept me. My breasts may be gone, replaced with implants, my right hand may swell with lymphedema, and I may have daily reminders of what cancer took—but I'm still here.

And I'm still becoming.

I still go to follow-up appointments. I still pause when a new ache or pain arises, wondering—*Is it back?* But I don't live in fear. I live in awareness. In deep gratitude. I've learned to be present with the now.

There are quiet moments when I watch my children laugh in another room, sit on the porch with a cup of coffee, or feel God's presence wash over me in prayer—and I think, *This is life. This is living.*

I'm not rushing anymore. I'm not trying to prove anything. I'm not performing for anyone's approval. I have peace now. And peace isn't loud—it doesn't need to be.

The woman who found a lump in the shower… she was scared. She was uncertain. She was keeping everything to herself, trying to carry it all.

But the woman writing this?

She knows the power of release.

She knows the beauty of asking for help.

She knows that healing is not just physical—it's emotional, mental, and spiritual.

She knows that sharing your story is part of your healing.

I've learned that cancer doesn't just interrupt your life—it rewrites it. But what I didn't expect was that God would use that rewriting to make something more meaningful than before. He didn't restore me to what I was. He rebuilt me into something new.

So if you're reading this and you're in the middle of your own fight—whether it's cancer or something else—I want you to know this:

You're not alone.

You are not forgotten.

And this is not the end of your story.

God still has a plan. There is purpose in your pain. And one day, you'll look back and see how far you've come—and you'll say, *I didn't just survive… I became.*

So walk in your new normal.

Speak up.

Love louder.

Rest when you need to.

Shine when you're ready.

Keep sharing your testimony, because your story is the blueprint for someone else's breakthrough.

And above all else—live, love, and BE authentic!

MEET THE AUTHORS

Meet Lisa!

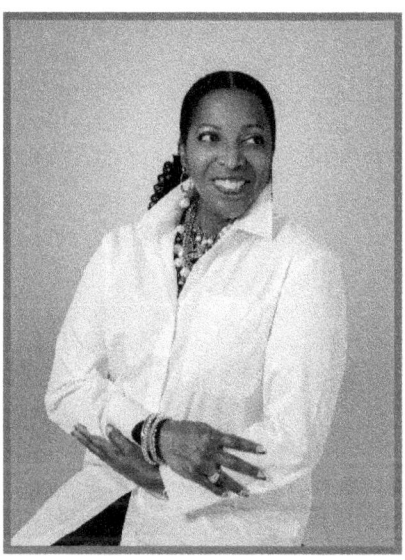

Lisa Gittens is a devoted wife, mother, and treasured friend whose life exemplifies the power of faith, service, and resilience. Her reputation precedes her, and her presence is a source of inspiration to many. Throughout her life, Lisa has dedicated her time and talents to supporting women and youth, empowering them to see their worth and embrace love, commitment, and sacrifice. She has instilled these values in her children, ensuring they understand the importance of giving back, and she continues to lead by example.

Lisa's unwavering dedication to service is made evident through her long-standing commitment to her church and community. From 1997 to 2015, she served as a praise and worship leader at LAM Christian Church, where she continues to be an active and vital member. Beyond the church walls, Lisa has served as a counselor at Naomi's Nest Drug Rehabilitation, offering guidance and support to those in recovery. Since 2018, Lisa has also devoted her time to prison ministry at Detroit Re-Entry and Huron Valley Women's Correctional Facility, providing hope and spiritual care to incarcerated women.

In 2021, Lisa faced a significant health challenge when she was diagnosed with mouth cancer. However, her faith and determination carried her through the ordeal, and by the grace of God, she overcame the illness. Lisa now shares her story as a powerful testament to the strength of resilience and faith. Her unwavering spirit continues to inspire those around her, and her life stands as a shining example of living with purpose, compassion, and a steadfast commitment to serving others.

Meet LaToya!

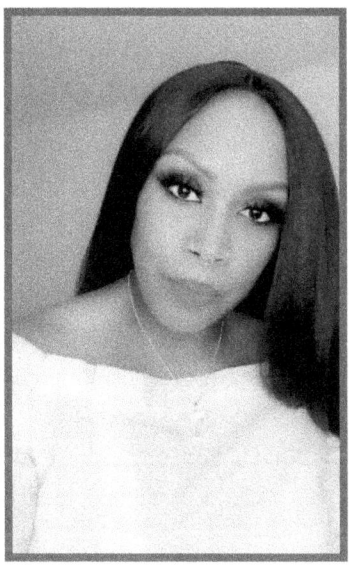

LaToya Murphy is a dynamic minister, educator, psalmist, and breast cancer survivor whose life and voice testify to the healing power of God. Born and raised in Franklin, VA, she is the youngest of four siblings and a proud daughter of Pastor Melvin and Lady Georgia Murphy. LaToya's love for gospel music began at the age of six in her father's church, and she's been singing ever since.

A licensed minister since 2012—the same year she was diagnosed with breast cancer—LaToya continued to preach, praise, and persevere, trusting God as her Healer. She has now been cancer-free for 13 years and serves faithfully as the Minister of Worship at Zion Baptist Church, Newport News, under the leadership of Dr. Tremayne M. Johnson.

LaToya has spent over 20 years in public education, currently serving as a Title I Liaison, which she considers an extension of her ministry. She holds two Bachelor's degrees from Virginia State University, is a 27-year member of Delta Sigma Theta Sorority, Inc., and has held licensure in mental health and human services (QMHP, QIDP, QMPP, CSS).

Known across the Hampton Roads region and beyond for her powerful voice and heartfelt worship, LaToya has sung with legendary gospel artists including Dorothy Norwood, Twinkie Clark, Donnie McClurkin, Yolanda Adams, Kirk Franklin, LeAndria Johnson, and more. She has recorded background vocals, appeared on Bobby Jones Gospel, and was a finalist in Sunday Best Season 7 auditions.

LaToya is the host of "The Healing Connection" podcast, "Manifestation Monday," and the Impact the Temple Exercise Program—all focused on holistic healing through the Word of God.

She is a proud mother of two adult children, Armani and Steven II, affectionately known as her "two blessings." In her spare time, she enjoys baking homemade pound cakes, braiding hair, piercing ears, and volunteering wherever there's a need.

A graduate of KC's Bible School and Education Program under Bishop Dr. Andrea Hall-Leonard, LaToya recently added co-author to her list of accomplishments.

Her life and ministry are anchored in Philippians 4:13: *"I can do everything through Him who gives me strength."*

Meet Judy!

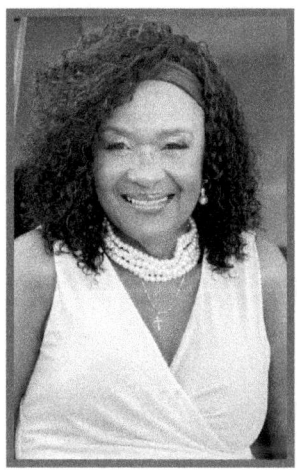

Judy Eve Lawrence-Lamb is a New York native and long-time Virginia resident who now resides in Charlotte, NC, with her family. A stage four metastatic breast cancer survivor, Judy has also overcome multiple strokes, single parenthood, domestic violence, and profound loss, yet her resilience and faith have remained unshaken.

A passionate writer, educator, and evangelist, Judy has authored multiple books, poetry, lyrics, and stage plays. She has worked as a correspondent writer, substitute teacher, and developmental editor at Tucker Publishing House, LLC. She is also the CEO of Wesleys & Eves Corporation—Un-ERASED and the beloved Grandma Judy Eve, bringing literacy programs to children.

Judy holds a BS in English from Norfolk State University and an M.Div. from Norfolk Theological Seminary & College. Called to ministry at 45, she obediently preached her initial sermon at 60.

Through her life's work, Judy inspires others to embrace their voice, overcome adversity, and trust in God's timing.

Email: healedone59@yahoo.com
Website: judywrites.com
YouTube: Grandma Judy Eve Productions (@grandmajudeve)

Meet Nicole!

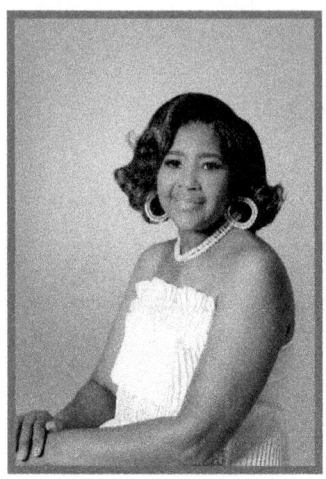

Nicole Dejo Lee, MA, LLPC, is a licensed mental health therapist, intercessor, and cancer survivor based in Flint, Michigan. With a deep passion for listening, encouraging, and uplifting others, Nicole lives out her God-given purpose daily through counseling and ministry.

She is the founder and CEO of Purlife Counseling Services, where she provides compassionate therapy with a focus on emotional healing, faith integration, and personal growth. Before stepping fully into the counseling field, Nicole served others faithfully for over 16 years as a funeral counselor, chaplain, and spent 8 years as a patient relations manager and customer service specialist in healthcare.

Nicole holds a Master's Degree in Clinical Counseling from Spring Arbor University and a Bachelor's Degree in Health Care Administration. Her approach to care is shaped not only by education and experience but also by personal healing—having survived cancer and openly sharing her testimony of God's miraculous power.

She is active in ministry and prayer, serving as:

- Moderator of Monday Morning Glory 6AM Prayer at New Jerusalem Full Gospel Baptist Church

MEET THE AUTHORS

- A leader with United Sisters, a ministry of healing and deliverance through storytelling
- A watchman intercessor with the Watchman Warrior Prayer Ministry
- A prayer leader and mentor with Chosen by God Ministry

Nicole has been featured on Chenelle Dismond's "Navigating Cancer" Facebook Live, shared her testimony at the Pink Night Palooza cancer event, and will be featured in a future Daily Bread devotional about the miraculous healing power of God.

Outside of her professional and ministry work, Nicole is a proud mother to her son, Colonel (Amber) Lee, a loving dog-mom to rescue pup Luna and granddog Mason. Known for her warmth, wisdom, and servant heart, Nicole remains committed to helping others find peace, purpose, and healing—both clinically and spiritually.

Meet Via!

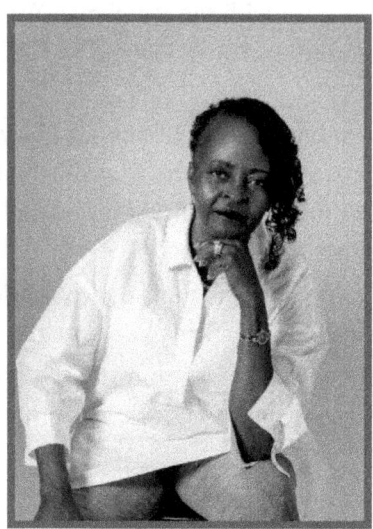

Vianessa "Via" Shephard is an accomplished HR Consultant with expertise in human resources management and client relations. She currently serves at a major utility company in Detroit, Michigan, where her passion for people, policy, and purpose drives her work.

Born and raised in Detroit, Via is deeply connected to her community and brings a personal touch to every professional space she enters. She holds a Bachelor's degree in Business Administration from the Detroit College of Business (now Davenport University) and a Master's degree in Industrial Relations from Wayne State University.

Via is a 14-year breast cancer survivor, and her journey through diagnosis, treatment, and healing is a powerful testimony of faith, resilience, and perseverance. Her experience informs her compassionate leadership style, making her a powerful advocate for supportive workplace culture and mental wellness.

She is an active member of LAM Christian Church, where she faithfully serves as an adjutant and co-leader of the women's ministry. Her love for God, community, and family is at the heart of everything she does.

MEET THE AUTHORS

Via and her husband Stan reside in Clinton Township, MI, and are proud parents of 10 children, 10 grandchildren, and 2 great-grandchildren. Together, they raise their three youngest children: Johnathan (19), MaKiya (15), and Jordan (12).

Beyond work and ministry, Via finds peace and inspiration in music, and enjoys therapeutic creative hobbies like paint-by-number art. She treasures time with her family and friends, valuing connection as a key to healing and joy.

Vianessa Shephard's story is one of strength, faith, and grace. She continues to inspire others by living a life rooted in purpose, love, and service.

Meet Marisa!

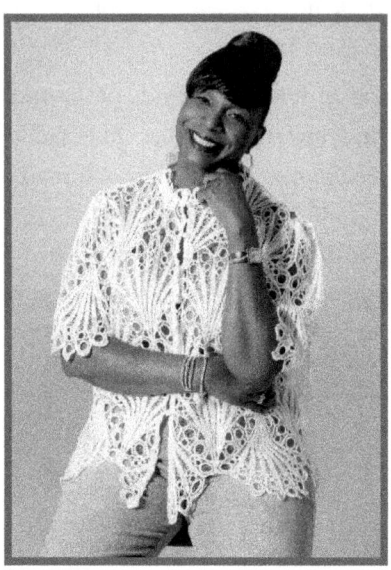

Marisa Youngblood, LMSW, CAADC, is a licensed clinical social worker, certified advanced alcohol and drug counselor. A breast and liver cancer survivor who continues to live with joy and purpose through God's guidance. A devoted wife, mother, and grandmother, Marisa is also hearing impaired and leads her life with strength, faith, and a commitment to helping others thrive despite adversity.

After over 30 years of service in the mental health and substance abuse fields, Marisa retired following her diagnosis of Invasive Ductal Carcinoma (HER2+ Positive) in 2020. During her tenure, she provided prevention and clinical counseling services for children, adolescents, and adults—including trauma-informed treatment, intensive home-based therapy, clinical supervision, and substance use recovery.

Today, Marisa serves as the Founder and Director of Life Changing Counseling Services, L.L.C., where she offers counseling, education, and life skills development for youth, families, and individuals dealing with trauma, addiction, and emotional struggles. Her practice emphasizes value systems, self-awareness, coping strategies, and healing through informed care.

Marisa is also a peer support volunteer with the American Cancer Society and supports women across the nation navigating breast cancer diagnoses. She is an active member of several advocacy and survivor networks including:

- Sisters Network of River Rouge
- Gilda's Club
- Taking Our Lives Back
- Black Women Surviving Survivorship Anthology
- My Sistah's Pink Journey
- LIFT After Breast Cancer
- The Transparency Table, Your Story Matters Here

She regularly joins cancer research with Karmanos Cancer Center and Wayne State University, participating in programs like C.A.P.A.B.L.E. and LIVESTRONG at the YMCA.

Active in her community and church, Marisa volunteers as a Behavioral Health Coordinator and serves on multiple boards for trauma-informed care and substance abuse prevention.

She provides behavioral health resources in Southfield and supports Detroit's Brightmoor community through Leland Missionary Baptist Church/Leland Community Affairs, Inc., and works with her District and State Ministries. She is a member of the National Association of Social Workers (NASW).

At 61, Marisa found her father and paternal relatives through Ancestry DNA, broadening her support network.

Her daily life is inspired by Isaiah 40:31 and Psalm 121:1–2.

Marisa walks over 10,000 steps each day and joins multiple fundraising walks annually.

Meet Sabrina!

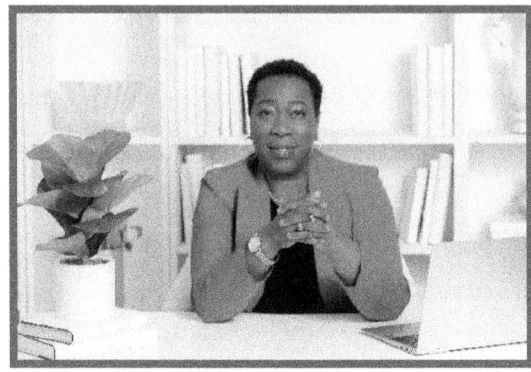

Sabrina Thomas is a Best-Selling Author, Speaker, Advocate, Breast Cancer Warrior, TV Producer with Zondra TV Network and a caregiver.

With over 20 years of experience as an advocate she has become a strong voice in the special needs community. Hoping to broaden the scope of her work and in line with her vision--she has started an empowerment community called "Girl Don't Count Yourself Out".

This community aims to connect women from all facets of life to focus on self-care, confidence and building self-worth. With this movement, Sabrina continues to follow her passion for service by supporting women while they step into becoming the most empowered and uplifted version of themselves. Sabrina openly and readily shares her life and career lessons with her audience and individual clients so they can learn from what worked and what did not work along her personal journey. Her ability to overcome obstacles, both professional and personal, has fueled her to stay-the-course to be successful in all her endeavors.

Today, Sabrina holds certifications in Advocacy, IEP Master Coaching, Speaker Training, as well as a Life Coach certification. Sabrina has numerous awards and has been in numerous magazines and has graced numerous magazine covers. Being an established author, Sabrina has co-written 18 books and is a 16-time Amazon Best Seller. In October 2021, she created along with her son but for him a coloring book series entitled "Color with Omar". These coloring books are a fun learning coloring experience where you get to learn about the creator (Omar) her special needs son in each series.

Meet Renee!

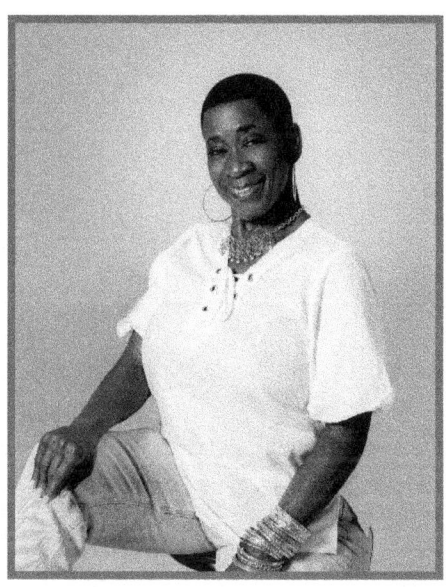

Renee M. Conley MA, SCL, LLPC, is an educator and has been a school counselor for the past 13 years. Renee currently works as the school counselor at DPSCD in Detroit, Michigan. She has been at Emerson elementary/middle school for the past 7 years. Before transferring back to DPSCD she was a High School Counselor at the Ypsilanti Community School District where she founded the ACCE Food Pantry, and she ran the Alternative School for High Schoolers. Renee completed her Masters' degree at the University of Detroit Mercy. Renee also works as a Mental Health therapist at Community Outreach for Psychiatric Emergencies/ Hegira Health INC. Renee volunteers monthly with her family to feed the homeless, she also founded the DPSCD Emerson Food Pantry. Renee can be found volunteering and participating in community service with her colleagues, as well as her students.' Renee is an advocate for students/families with mental health issues who need help navigating/transitioning to high school and/or college. Renee is also the proud business owner of PHAT Girlz Heavyn LLC. Renee is a professional vocalist who sings gospel, jazz, and R/B, abroad and across the US. Renee is currently working on her new CD. It will be available soon.

Meet Monica!

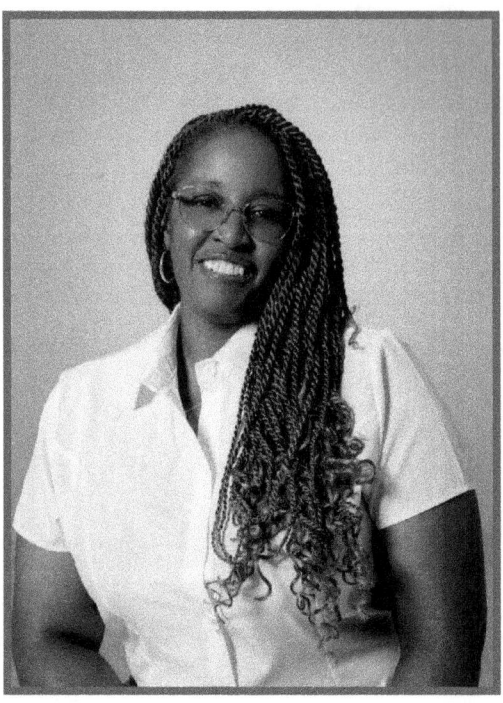

Monica Poe is a proud mom of three miracle babies, a survivor, a creator, and a woman of unshakable faith. A high school graduate and former employee of FCA (Fiat Chrysler Automobiles), Monica is currently a stay-at-home mom who finds joy in crafting—pouring her love into handmade creations that brighten the lives of others.

Her chapter in Surviving Survivorship Anthology marks her powerful debut as an author. In it, she opens her heart to share a journey of profound loss, resilience, and unwavering faith. Monica has experienced more than most—she has survived 26 miscarriages, stage 2 breast cancer, a full hysterectomy, and a double mastectomy. Today, she is celebrating two years cancer-free and continues to walk in gratitude and strength.

Monica is a woman of prayer and purpose. As a member of Jewels Ladies of Prayer, she finds strength in sisterhood and devotion. Though life has brought immense challenges, including the loss of her beloved mother to breast cancer at just 48, Monica remains grounded in faith, always willing to share her testimony with anyone who will listen.

After 33 years in a relationship—16 of those married—Monica is now navigating a new chapter of self-discovery and healing while co-parenting with grace. An only child herself, she is a natural listener and a source of wisdom and comfort to those around her. She is a woman with many ideas, a heart full of compassion, and a spirit ready to inspire others on their own paths of survival and self-love.

Meet Neicy!

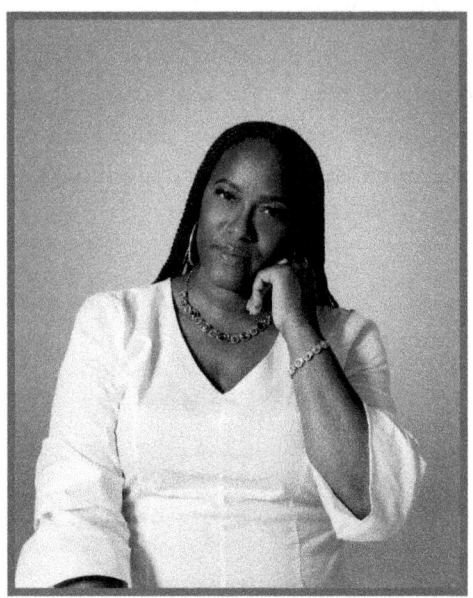

Nosalind "Neicy" Johnson is the founder and President of Taking Our Lives Back of Michigan. A proud Detroit native, she graduated from Mumford High School and is a devoted mother of two and grandmother of two. With over 29 years of experience as a Customer Experience Operator at a publishing company, Neicy also spent more than a decade on the fundraising team, personally leading numerous successful events and initiatives.

Beyond her professional achievements, Neicy is deeply committed to giving back to her community. She has volunteered with various organizations including Habitat for Humanity, the Life Remodeled Project, and the Oasis Men's Shelter. She has also distributed "blessing bags" to the homeless in Detroit and served on the boards of WROSES and The Elite Women Organization, where she led the Event Team for three years. She currently serves as Board Secretary for Reece World of Michigan.

In March 2004, Neicy received a life-altering diagnosis: stage 3B Hodgkin's Lymphoma. Despite the cancer's high survival rate, it had already spread to her neck, underarms, chest, and lungs. With her children just 13 and 5 years old at the time, she made the immediate decision to begin chemotherapy. Though surrounded by support from family and friends, she couldn't stop thinking about the women battling cancer without a similar support system.

By September 2004, Neicy was declared cancer-free, completing her final round of chemotherapy the following month, in October. However, even during her recovery, she felt a greater calling to help others fighting the same battle. In 2006, she began with small steps—participating in cancer walks, donating to various organizations, and purchasing items that contributed proceeds toward cancer causes. Still, she knew in her heart that she could do more.

That vision became clearer when she came across a breast cancer survivor calendar. She was captivated by the idea: showcasing women currently battling cancer—and survivors—while allowing them to share their stories and be celebrated. Inspired, Neicy began planning. After years of research and preparation, she launched the first Taking Our Lives Back calendar in 2013. Its mission was simple but profound: to give women a day of pampering—including makeup, a photoshoot, and the chance to tell their story. The calendar became a beacon of hope, designed to encourage other women to keep fighting and not give up, even through the hardships of chemotherapy, hair loss, surgeries, radiation, pain, and depression.

A portion of the proceeds from calendar sales has been donated to impactful organizations, including The Barbara Ann Karmanos Cancer Institute, Lymphoma Research Foundation, Josephine Ford Cancer Center, Cancer Awareness and Resource Network, and My Sistah's Pink Journey. These organizations help cancer patients and their families with essential needs like living expenses and resources for care.

In October 2024, Nosalind celebrated 20 years cancer-free, a milestone that stands as a testament to her strength and faith. Through her organization, she continues to produce empowering calendars featuring women who are either surviving or currently fighting cancer. She also creates and distributes chemo care packages to women undergoing active treatment—small but meaningful tokens of hope and encouragement.

Nosalind's journey is one of faith, purpose, and unwavering service. In addition to her advocacy work, she enjoys dancing, traveling, and spending quality time with her family and friends.

Meet Valerie!

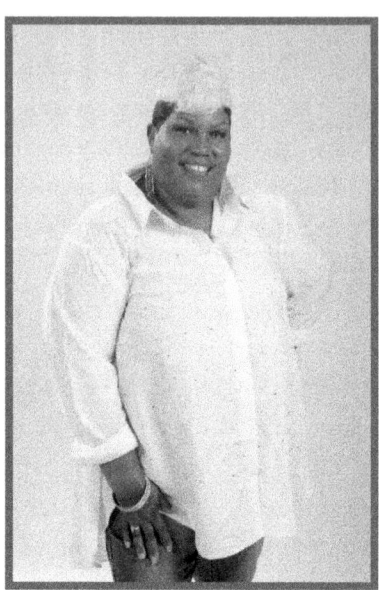

Valerie Wilder is a devoted daughter of the Most High God and a woman gifted with the Holy Spirit-led gift of Exhortation. She is a wife of 44 years, proud mother of three, and grandmother of eight—a role she treasures deeply.

After a fulfilling 43-year career in the Healthcare Industry, Valerie recently retired, having served as a Medical Receptionist, Medical Transcriptionist, Supervisor, and Training Coordinator. Her work was marked by excellence in customer service, emotional intelligence, team building, and compassionate communication. She now seeks to empower other healthcare professionals through her business by equipping them with these same skills to make a meaningful impact in patient care.

As a certified Emotional Intelligence Practitioner, Valerie is passionate about helping others—especially youth—understand and manage their emotions in a way that honors God's design. Her heart's desire is to guide young people toward wise decision-making and a life aligned with God's purpose, rather than being led by destructive emotional patterns.

Valerie's creative side shines through her love of journaling, writing poetry, and dancing. Her earlier years included dancing on the Norfolk-based TV show *Calvin Shakespear and the Get Down People*, earning the title of Ms.

Congeniality in Hal Jackson's Talented Teens (1975), and serving as President of the Hospitality Ministry at First Pentecostal Church.

Valerie's testimony is one of incredible resilience. She has overcome bullying, mental health struggles, breast cancer, other health challenges, and most recently, the devastating loss of her son in 2023. Through it all, God has kept her, strengthened her, and positioned her to comfort and encourage others walking through seasons of deep pain and uncertainty.

Her life reflects a powerful truth: God can heal, restore, and use every part of our story for His glory.

Meet Sandra!

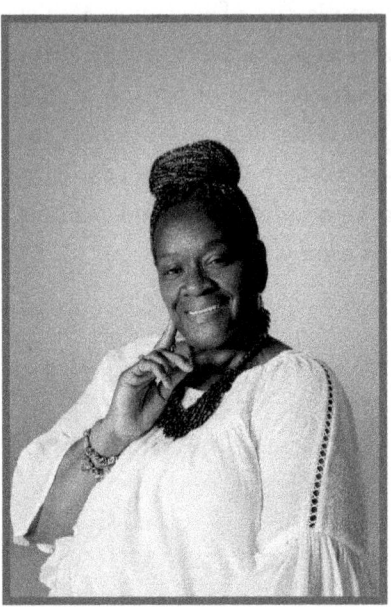

Sandra Marie Ewing is a resilient woman of strength and compassion, proudly residing in Holt, Michigan. A retired employee of the City of Lansing, Sandra is a devoted mother of four, grandmother of fifteen, and great-grandmother of three. Her life is a testament to endurance, faith, and a deep desire to serve others.

Sandra has survived breast cancer three times, and she now walks boldly in her calling to support others on similar journeys. Her greatest passion is helping individuals battling cancer stay strong, keep their faith, and navigate the often-overwhelming world of treatment, recovery, and resources. She lovingly offers guidance, emotional support, and directs those in need to helpful services—doing all she can to be a light in their darkest moments.

In her personal life, Sandra enjoys walking, watching movies, and spending quiet moments in journaling, which has become one of her favorite forms of reflection and healing. She believes in the power of connection, encouragement, and honest conversations that uplift the soul.

Sandra's story is one of survival, faith, and purpose—and her mission is clear: to ensure no one walks through cancer alone.

Meet Tara!

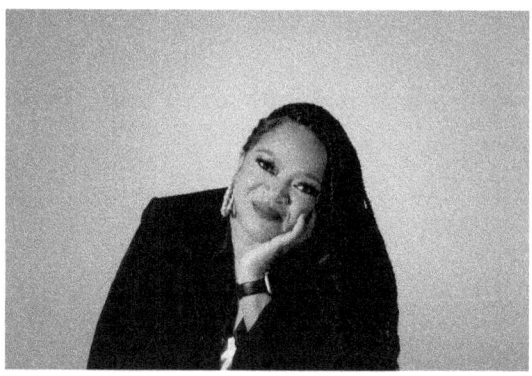

Tara Tucker is a best-selling author, certified life coach, certified solution-focused coach, and behavioral science professional. She is also a dynamic storyteller, innovative strategist, and faith-driven mentor. As a daughter of the Most-High God, Tara wears many hats—book and life coach, publisher, podcast host, workshop facilitator, and marketplace minister.

She is the founder and CEO of Tucker Publishing House, LLC, where she helps authors bring powerful, purpose-filled books to life. Tara is also the visionary behind Jewels Ladies of Prayer Outreach, an intercessory prayer group, and Her Authentic Voice, a global faith-based initiative and podcast that explores healing, identity, and the power of testimony.

Tara holds associate degrees in Pre-Psychology and the Arts, along with a Behavioral Science Certification from Macomb Community College. With over a decade of experience in coaching and consulting, she combines biblical wisdom, emotional intelligence, and personal testimony to help others grow, heal, and lead.

A survivor of childhood trauma, stage 3 breast cancer, and sepsis shock, Tara openly shares her journey to offer strength and remind others that their testimony is someone else's breakthrough. Her impactful work has been featured on iHeart Radio's Monica Morgan Speaks, Canvas Rebel, and The Michigan Chronicle.

Tara is deeply committed to youth empowerment. She has mentored youth through The IMAGINE Mentoring Program of Michigan and Citadel of Perpetual **Learning**, and she has facilitated numerous writing workshops—

including the Prepare & Publish Youth Writing Workshops based on her children's book, "I'm Not Too Little to Write a Book and Neither Are You."

Through her writing, coaching, and publishing programs, Tara empowers faith-driven women to embrace their voices, heal from within, and publish with purpose. She lives by her personal motto: **liveloveBEauthentic**, committed to authentic living, spiritual growth, and building real connections.

Epilogue: Your Story Continues

Sister, you made it to the end. But this isn't really the end, is it? This is where your story begins.

You've just witnessed something sacred—women who chose to be transparent with their pain so you could find strength for your own journey. Each testimony you've read cost something. Each story required courage to tell. And some of these voices... some of them we almost lost in the telling.

Let me be honest with you about what it took to bring these stories to your hands.

This was an uphill battle to write and release. While we were collecting testimonies of triumph, the battle was still raging for some of our contributors. Ms. Kaye—Romana Kaye Simons—passed away before we had a chance to hear her story. Her voice was silenced before she could add it to this collection, and that loss still sits heavy on my heart.

Nicole wrote her beautiful story of resilience and faith. She was radiant, faith-filled, a warrior in every sense of the word. But during the process of book production, cancer returned more aggressively, and we lost her too. Her chapter stands as a monument to her courage, but knowing she won't see the impact of her words—that breaks something in you.

Marisa Youngblood's cancer returned while we were working on this anthology. But Marisa? She beat it AGAIN. She's a survivor yet again, and she was able to add her new testimony to her chapter. That woman is unstoppable.

Renee Conley was receiving treatment but on the tail end of it as we compiled these stories. Sandra Ewing was facing cancer's return, fighting battles we couldn't see while sharing her strength with you.

You see, Sister, while you were reading about victory, some of our contributors were still in the valley. While you were being inspired by their faith, they were living it out in real time—doctor appointments, treatments, uncertainty, and pain.

This anthology exists because women decided their stories mattered more than their comfort. Because they believed YOUR breakthrough was worth their transparency.

> *"Therefore encourage one another and build each other up, just as in fact you are doing."*
> **- 1 Thessalonians 5:11 (ESV)**

So here's what I need you to understand as you close this book: You carry their legacy now. You carry Romana's unspoken story. You carry Nicole's unfinished dreams. You carry the courage of every woman who bled on these pages so you could find healing.

Their testimonies weren't given to entertain you—they were given to equip you. Their transparency wasn't for applause—it was for your advancement. Their vulnerability wasn't weakness—it was warfare against the shame, silence, and self-doubt that's been keeping you small.

What are you going to DO with what you've received?

Because receiving these stories without responding to them is like accepting a gift and never unwrapping it. Like being handed keys to freedom and choosing to stay locked up. Like having a testimony and keeping it to yourself when someone else is drowning in the very waters you survived.

You have work to do, Sister.

You have healing to walk in. You have truth to speak. You have authenticity to embrace. You have a voice that's been waiting for permission to be heard.

The women in this book didn't fight their battles so you could stay comfortable. They didn't share their scars so you could hide yours. They didn't break their silence so you could keep yours.

Some of them are no longer here to encourage you in person. Some of them are still fighting battles you can't see. But ALL of them believed in your potential to overcome, to thrive, to become who God created you to be.

Their sacrifice demands your stewardship.

So as you walk away from this anthology, remember: You're not just inspired—you're equipped. You're not just encouraged—you're expected. Expected to take what you've learned and let it transform how you live.

EPILOGUE: YOUR STORY CONTINUES

Stop playing small. Stop hiding your story. Stop believing the lie that your mess disqualifies you from ministry, that your struggles make you unworthy of success, that your scars make you less than beautiful.

These women fought cancer, betrayal, loss, rejection, fear—and WON. They didn't win because they were special. They won because they refused to stay down. Because they chose faith over fear, truth over lies, authenticity over approval.

You can do the same.

Your story isn't over. Your best chapters haven't been written yet. Your greatest victory might be waiting on the other side of your current challenge.

But you have to choose it. You have to fight for it. You have to believe you're worth the battle.

In the back of this book, you'll find resources to help you on your journey. Use them. Don't just collect inspiration—take action. Don't just feel motivated—get moving.

And remember—you're not walking this path alone. Every woman in this anthology is cheering you on from wherever they are. They're praying for your breakthrough, believing in your potential, knowing that their stories will find purpose in your transformation.

Live loud, Sister. Love hard. BE authentic.

Your voice matters. Your story matters. YOU matter.

And your greatest chapter is still being written.

Go write it.

With fierce faith, an unshakeable belief in your destiny, and many blessings,

Coach Tara
Your favorite Shift Your Story Coach
#liveloveBEauthentic

RESOURCE

New Day Foundation

New Day Foundation for Families provides financial and emotional resources to Michigan families facing cancer.
    https://www.foundationforfamilies.org/who-we-are/

Share a Smile

Share A Smile is a Michigan-based charitable organization founded in 1999 to meet the needs of ordinary citizens struggling with financial crises due to unemployment, health crises, or natural disasters. For additional information, visit their website at www.Shareasmile.org or call (248) 792-9406.

Family Reach

Family Reach provides immediate assistance, education, and outreach to qualified families through financial grants that directly help families in need. For additional information, visit their website at www.familyreach.org or call (973) 394-1411

A Mother's Wish

A Mother's Wish embraces and supports Oakland County, MI, women and families impacted by breast cancer by easing the day-to-day burdens associated with a diagnosis while offering opportunities for hope, comfort, family togetherness, and healing. For additional information, visit their website at www.amotherswishmichigan.com or email contactus@amotherswishmichigan.com

Angels of Hope

Angels of Hope is a Non-Profit Organization founded in 2004 that offers financial assistance, volunteer teachers, portraits, and holiday programs to families affected by Cancer. For additional information, visit their website at www.angelsofhope.org or call (586) 226-3146.

The Pink Fund

The Pink Fund is a Non-Profit Organization founded in 2007 that offers up to 90 days of non-medical financial aid to cover basic cost-of-living expenses for breast cancer patients who have lost all or part of their income during active treatment. For additional information, visit their website at http://pinkfund.org/ or call (877) 234-PINK (7465).

The Sam Fund

The Sam Fund is a Non-Profit Organization founded in 2003 that offers financial assistance and free online support and education to young adult cancer survivors. For additional information, visit their website at www.thesamfund.org or call (617) 938-3484.

Cancer Treatment Centers of America

The Cancer Treatment Centers of America is a Private, for-profit operator of cancer treatment hospitals and outpatient clinics founded in 1988 that uses leading technology to aggressively treat cancer. They also support their patients with nutrition and other therapies, because they recognize that managing the side effects of cancer treatment is half the battle. For additional information, visit their website at www.cancercenter.com or call (800) 931-0599.

Cleaning for a Reason

Cleaning for a Reason is a non-profit organization founded in 2006 that offers professional house cleaning to women experiencing cancer. For additional information, visit their website at www.cleaningforareason.org or call (877) 337-3348.

Camp Kesem

The Camp Kesum is a Non-Profit Organization founded in 2000 that offers week-long summer camps catered explicitly to children between the ages of 6 and 16 with a parent affected by cancer. For additional information, visit their website at http://campkesem.org/msu or call (502) 430-2267.

Look Good Feel Better

The Look Good Feel Better is a Non-Profit Organization founded in 1989 that offers Tips for Teens, Men, and Women affected by cancer. Workshops for 2-hour women, hands-on workshops that include: A detailed description and demonstration of the 12-step skin care and makeup program, Instruction on options relating to hair loss, including wigs (types/care), turbans, and scarves, nail care and helpful suggestions on clothing and ways to use flattering colors and shapes, as well as ways to camouflage areas of concern during cancer treatment. For additional information, visit their website at http://lookgoodfeelbetter.org/ or call (800) 395-LOOK.

Emotional Support

Imerman Angels

The Imerman Angels is a Non-Profit Organization founded in 2003 that matches those affected by cancer with a cancer survivor or survivor's caregiver who is the same age, same gender, and most importantly, who has faced the same type of cancer. For additional information, visit their website at http://www.imermanangels.org/ or call (877) 274-5529.

Gilda's Club

Gilda's Club is a Non-Profit Organization founded in 1998 that offers support groups, education lectures, workshops, children/teen-specific activities and groups, bereavement support groups, and social events for men, women, teens, and children living with cancer, as well as their families and friends. For additional information, visit their website at www.gildasclubdetroit.org or call (248) 577-0800.

The Lake House

The Lake House is a Non-Profit Organization founded in 2011 that offers cancer support groups, one-on-one cancer support consultations/guidance, health and wellness talks/activities, stress management activities, and social events to those affected by cancer in Northeast Wayne County and Macomb County. For additional information, visit their website at milakehouse.org or call (586) 777-7761.

Retreats

Memories of Love

The Memories of Love is a Non-Profit Organization founded in 2005 that offers vacations to parents with a life-threatening diagnosis and children under the age of 16. Trips included 5-night, 6-day vacations in Orlando, including 3-day passes for the wish recipient and their children, a 1-day pass to SeaWorld, and a 2-day pass to Universal Studios. Also included are hotel accommodations, discount meal vouchers (based on availability) at select restaurants, and $100 to help defray the cost of food, gas, parking, etc. For additional information, visit their website at www.memoriesoflove.org or call (904) 596-2789.

Little Pink Houses of Hope

Little Pink Houses of Hope is a non-profit organization founded in 2010 that offers week-long vacation retreats for breast cancer patients and their families. For additional information, visit their website at https://littlepink.org/ or call (336) 213-4733.

Inheritance of Hope

The Inheritance of Hope is a non-profit organization founded in 2007 that offers legacy retreats, scholarship resources, book resources, continuing support post-retreat, and webinars to families consisting of children under 18 years of age and a parent with a life-threatening illness (Cancer Stages 3 or 4).

For additional information, visit their website at http://inheritanceofhope.org/ or call (914) 213-8435.

Additional Websites

- http://www.patientresource.com/Financial_Resources.aspx
- http://www.cancer.gov/cancertopics/aya/resources
- http://www.needymeds.org

1. Hover over "Patient Savings."
2. Click on "Diagnosis-Based Assistance."
3. Click on "By Diagnosis."
4. Find the diagnosis, Select It
5. Scroll down to see resources, being careful to check what region----- support is offered in by checking the far right-hand column

If you want to share your story in the next volume, scan the QR code below.

www.ingramcontent.com/pod-product-compliance
Lightning Source LLC
Chambersburg PA
CBHW050902160426
43194CB00011B/2251